Profiles of Early Expressive Phonological Skills™ (PEEPS™)

Examiner's Manual

Profiles of Early Expressive Phonological Skills™ (PEEPS™)

Examiner's Manual

by

A. Lynn Williams, Ph.D.
East Tennessee State University
Johnson City

and

Carol Stoel-Gammon, Ph.D.
University of Washington
Seattle

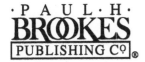

·P A U L·H·
BROOKES
PUBLISHING Co.®

Baltimore • London • Sydney

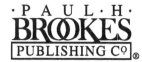

Paul H. Brookes Publishing Co.
Post Office Box 10624
Baltimore, Maryland 21285-0624
USA

www.brookespublishing.com

Typeset by Progressive Publishing Services, York, Pennsylvania.
Manufactured in the United States of America by
Integrated Books International, Inc., Dulles, Virginia.

The individuals described in this book are composites or real people whose situations are masked
and are based on the authors' experiences. In all instances, names and identifying details have been
changed to protect confidentiality.

This manual accompanies the Profiles of Early Expressive Phonological Skills™ (PEEPS™). The PEEPS
Test Forms are available for separate purchase in packages of ten. To learn more or to place an online
order, please visit https://brookespublishing.com/product/PEEPS.

Library of Congress Cataloging-in-Publication Data

Names: Williams, A. Lynn, author. | Stoel-Gammon, Carol, author.
Title: Profiles of Early Expressive Phonological Skills (PEEPS) examiner's manual / by A. Lynn Williams
  and Carol Stoel-Gammon.
Description: Baltimore : Paul H. Brookes Publishing Co., 2023. | Includes bibliographical references
  and index.
Identifiers: LCCN 2022051228 | ISBN 9781681257389 (paperback)
Subjects: LCSH: Profiles of Early Expressive Phonological Skills (Test) | English language—
  Phonology—Ability testing. | Children—Language—Testing.
Classification: LCC LB1139.L3 W486 2023 | DDC 372.6/044—dc23/eng/20221209
LC record available at https://lccn.loc.gov/2022051228

British Library Cataloguing in Publication data are available from the British Library.

2027   2026   2025   2024   2023

10   9   8   7   6   5   4   3   2   1

Contents

About the Video

Visit the Brookes Download Hub to stream an illustrative video that demonstrates how the *Profiles of Early Expressive Phonological Skills*™ (*PEEPS*™) assessment is administered. In the PEEPS Demonstration Video, several clinicians administer the PEEPS to young children; the examiners demonstrate the elicitation procedures and other important practices for administration.

Purchasers of this book may stream and view the video for professional and educational use. To access the materials that come with this book:

1. Go to the Brookes Download Hub: http://downloads.brookespublishing.com

2. Register to create an account (or log in with an existing account)

3. Redeem the code **TvbnsyvJK** to access any locked materials

About the Authors

A. Lynn Williams, Ph.D., Interim Dean and Professor, East Tennessee State University, Johnson City

Lynn Williams is Interim Dean in the College of Clinical and Rehabilitative Health Sciences and Professor in the Department of Audiology and Speech-Language Pathology at East Tennessee State University. Most of her research has involved clinical investigations of models of phonological treatment for children with severe to profound speech sound disorders. She developed a new model of phonological intervention called multiple oppositions that has been the basis of federally funded intervention studies by the National Institutes of Health (NIH) and developed a phonological intervention software program called Sound Contrasts in Phonology (SCIP) that was funded by NIH. Dr. Williams served as associate editor of *Language, Speech, and Hearing Services in the Schools* and the *American Journal of Speech-Language Pathology*. Dr. Williams is a Fellow of the American Speech-Language-Hearing Association and is currently serving as ASHA Immediate Past President (2021 ASHA President).

Carol Stoel-Gammon, Ph.D., Professor Emerita, Department of Speech and Hearing Sciences, University of Washington, Seattle

Carol Stoel-Gammon received her Ph.D. in linguistics with a specialization in developmental psycholinguistics from Stanford University in 1974. She is currently Professor Emerita in the Department of Speech and Hearing Sciences at the University of Washington in Seattle. During her career, she has taught linguistics in Brazil (Universidade Federal, Campinas, Brazil, 1974–1976) and at the University of Colorado, Boulder (1982–1984). Her research and publications have focused on cross-linguistic studies of phonological development, speech and language development in infants and toddlers with typical and atypical development, the relationship between babble and speech, and the relationship between early lexical and early phonological development. Dr. Stoel-Gammon has served as Associate Editor of the *Journal of Speech and Hearing Disorders*, the *Journal of Speech and Hearing Research* and the *American Journal of Speech-Language Pathology*. She became a Fellow of the American Speech-Language Hearing Association in 2005 and was awarded Honors of the Association in 2014.

ABOUT THE CONTRIBUTOR

Nancy J. Scherer, Ph.D., Professor, Department of Speech and Hearing Science, Arizona State University, Tempe

Dr. Nancy Scherer is a professor of speech and hearing science at Arizona State University. She conducts research on assessment and intervention efficacy for young children with craniofacial conditions. She focuses on assessing effectiveness of early intervention service delivery models (telehealth, parent training, and hybrid) for application in the United States and international contexts.

Foreword

During the first years of life, children are welcomed into families and communities and develop their sense of identity. Early childhood is the beginning of life's journey—to find joy, fulfilment, and purpose in society. Young children are important to society, now and in the future. Communication is a key to unlocking children's capacity to develop their identity, their connection with their family and community, their academic and social skills, and their future employment and citizenship. Article 12 of the Convention on the Rights of the Child states:

> States Parties shall assure to the child who is capable of forming his or her own views the right to express those views freely in all matters affecting the child, the views of the child being given due weight in accordance with the age and maturity of the child. . . . (United Nations, 1989)

Children need to be afforded the capacity to communicate, and people need to listen. Article 12 applies across the world, since 195 countries (United Nations States Parties) have signed this Convention. Assuring children the right to form and express their views is a two-way process. Communication typically involves *speaking* and *listening*—and communication is facilitated by intelligible communication.

Children begin vocalizing at birth, and they quickly begin to coo and babble. Around their first birthdays, they use some recognizable words. Between the ages of 18–36 months, children's capacity to speak and be understood explodes. Speech and language development interact (Stoel-Gammon, 2011). During this time, children develop three major components of speech within their ambient language: 1) segmental aspects of speech (i.e., individual phonemes), 2) phonotactic constraints and structures (i.e., how the segments relate to one another), and 3) suprasegmental or prosodic aspects of speech (i.e., pitch, intonation, stress, rhythm, and tones) (Stoel-Gammon & Peter, 2008). Most segmental and suprasegmental aspects are mastered early. In a review of children's consonant acquisition in 27 languages by 5 years of age, most children can produce most of the consonants in their ambient languages (McLeod & Crowe, 2018) and children are intelligible, even to strangers (McLeod, 2020). Phonotactic constraints and structures (e.g., consonant clusters, polysyllabic words) are learned concurrently but may take a little longer to master (Masso et al., 2017; McLeod et al., 2001).

To date, there have been few tools available to speech-language pathologists (SLPs) to assess young children's emerging speech skills. The Profiles of Early Expressive Phonological Skills™ (PEEPS) has been designed for young children (18–36 months of age) who have small vocabularies and limited inventories of speech sounds. PEEPS™ is a unique evidence-based speech assessment and is a welcome addition to SLPs' almost empty toolboxes for young children. The word list has been carefully selected using the authors' extensive knowledge of young children's vocabularies and emerging speech skills, and children can enjoy the process of naming toys during "play" (i.e., assessment). The PEEPS™ profile is a "multilayered description of a child's phonological system" (p. 5) that enables SLPs to gain an overview of children's strengths and identify "warning signs" or "red flags for phonetic and phonological development" (p. 68).

The authors of PEEPS™ are eminent authorities on children's speech and have undertaken extensive research that underpins their conceptualization and operationalization of this unique tool. They have spent more than 15 years developing PEEPS™, and the world has been waiting. PEEPS™ has proven value for working with young children, including those with cleft lip and palate (Scherer et al., 2012).

The speech-language pathology profession began with a strong focus on speech production. Children with speech sound disorders (SSD) represent one of the largest groups of pediatric clients (Mullen & Schooling, 2010). A comprehensive understanding of speech development forms the basis of SLPs' clinical decision making in the areas of assessment, diagnosis, selection of intervention targets and approaches, intervention, identification and prediction of outcomes, and timing of discharge from intervention (Williams et al., 2021). Early identification of warning signs for SSD is important for scheduling early intervention and prevention of long-term communication, literacy, educational, social, and occupational issues (McCormack et al., 2009). Decisions whether a child is a late talker and/ or has SSD (Hodges et al., 2022; Stoel-Gammon, 1991) present a challenge that requires a comprehensive assessment designed for a young child. Diagnostic speech information is a prerequisite for identification of SSD and facilitates clinical judgments regarding whether young children require speech intervention (Shriberg et al., 1994; To et al., 2022).

SLPs can learn a lot about young children's speech using PEEPS™ in order to make timely evidence-based decisions regarding early intervention. PEEPS™ can be used by SLPs to support young children's communication skills at the beginning of life's journey, so that through life's journey they have communicative competence to find purpose, fulfilment, and joy.

Sharynne McLeod, Ph.D., CPSP, Life Member SPA, ASHA Honors
Charles Sturt University, Australia

REFERENCES

Hodges, R., Baker, E., Munro, N., & Masso, S. (2022). The emergent literacy skills of 4- to 5-year-old children with and without a history of late talking. *International Journal of Speech-Language Pathology*, Advance online publication. https://doi.org/10.1080/17549507.2022.2152866

Masso, S., Baker, E., McLeod, S., & Wang, C. (2017). Polysyllable speech accuracy and predictors of later literacy development in preschool children with speech sound disorders. *Journal of Speech, Language, and Hearing Research, 60*(7), 1877–1890. https://doi.org/10.1044/2017_JSLHR-S-16-0171

McCormack, J., McLeod, S., McAllister, L., & Harrison, L. J. (2009). A systematic review of the association between childhood speech impairment and participation across the lifespan. *International Journal of Speech-Language Pathology, 11*, 155–170. https://doi.org/10.1080/17549500802676859

McLeod, S. (2020). Intelligibility in Context Scale: Cross-linguistic use, validity, and reliability. *Speech, Language and Hearing, 23*(1), 9–16. https://doi.org/10.1080/2050571X.2020.1718837

McLeod, S., & Crowe, K. (2018). Children's consonant acquisition in 27 languages: A cross-linguistic review. *American Journal of Speech-Language Pathology, 27*(4), 1546–1571. https://doi.org/10.1044/2018_AJSLP-17-0100

McLeod, S., van Doorn, J., & Reed, V. A. (2001). Normal acquisition of consonant clusters. *American Journal of Speech-Language Pathology, 10*, 99–110. https://doi.org/10.1044/1058-0360(2001/011)

Mullen, R., & Schooling, T. (2010). The National Outcomes Measurement System for pediatric speech-language pathology. *Language, Speech, and Hearing Services in Schools, 41*, 44–60. https://doi.org/10.1044/0161-1461(2009/08-0051)

Scherer, N. J., Williams, A. L., Stoel-Gammon, C., & Kaiser, A. (2012). Assessment of single-word production for children under three years of age: Comparison of children with and without cleft palate. *International Journal of Otolaryngology, 72*, 827–840. https://doi.org/10.1155/2012/724214

Shriberg, L. D., Kwiatkowski, J., & Gruber, F. A. (1994). Developmental phonological disorders II: Short-term speech-sound normalisation. *Journal of Speech and Hearing Research, 37*, 1127–1150. https://doi.org/10.1044/jshr.3705.1127

Stoel-Gammon, C. (1991). Normal and disordered phonology in two-year-olds. *Topics in Language Disorders, 11*, 21–32.

Stoel-Gammon, C. (2011). Relationships between lexical and phonological development in young children. *Journal of Child Language, 38*(1), 1–34. https://doi.org/10.1017/S0305000910000425

Stoel-Gammon, C., & Peter, B. (2008). Syllables, segments, and sequences: Phonological patterns in the words of young children acquiring American English. In B. L. Davis & K. Zajdo (Eds.), *The syllable in speech production* (pp. 293–323). Taylor & Francis. https://doi.org/10.4324/9780203837894

To, C. K. S., McLeod, S., Sam, K. L., & Law, T. (2022). Predicting which children will normalize without intervention for speech sound disorders. *Journal of Speech, Language, and Hearing Research, 65*(5), 1724–1741. https://doi.org/doi:10.1044/2022_JSLHR-21-00444

United Nations. (1989). *Convention on the rights of the child.* Retrieved from https://www.unicef.org/crc/

Williams, A. L., McLeod, S., & McCauley, R. J. (Eds.). (2021). *Interventions for speech sound disorders in children* (2nd ed.). Paul H. Brookes Publishing Co.

Preface

The idea for a developmentally appropriate assessment of early phonological skills has been part of the authors' clinical and research work for decades. In 1980, Carol and colleagues from the University of Washington received funding for a longitudinal study of 40 infants, ages 9–24 months, with the goal of assessing prelinguistic and early linguistic vocal and verbal development (Olswang, Stoel-Gammon, Coggins, & Carpenter, 1987, *Assessing Prelinguistic and Early Linguistic Behaviors in Developmentally Young Children*). The research team developed techniques for data collection using a variety of age-appropriate toys and props.

Lynn's doctoral work with Dr. Mary Elbert at Indiana University involved a longitudinal study of Late Talkers (LTs) using a bucket of toys that was considered to be more developmentally appropriate than asking toddlers to name illustrations (cf., Williams & Elbert, 2003). At that point, test words were selected that represented English consonants in word-initial and word-final positions that were easy to represent in common toys. Following that work years later, there was evidence that there was more to creating a developmentally appropriate assessment than the materials used to elicit the words. Part of Carol's extensive research on early lexical and phonological development involved completing phonetic analyses of the early acquired words from the MacArthur Communicative Developmental Inventories (CDIs; 1993; 2006). Working together, we have combined our clinical and research backgrounds in developing *Profiles of Early Expressive Phonological Skills*™ (*PEEPS*™), a developmentally appropriate assessment of toddlers' phonological skills.

Our aim in developing PEEPS was to provide speech-language pathologists and researchers with a developmentally appropriate assessment for toddlers (18–36 months) in identification of early phonological skills. There are a number of motivations for a developmentally appropriate test. For this young age group, there is a strong link between early lexical development and phonology, such that the two interact. Specifically, toddlers' phonological abilities are linked to the selection of words for early vocabulary. Secondly, phonological development is more closely associated with vocabulary size than with age. These two points indicate that phonological assessment of LTs and other children with limited vocabularies should not be based on traditional articulation tests. Instead, a test is needed that elicits words that are likely to be in the vocabulary of young children with typical development. Finally, early phonological development is more variable in children as a result of their acquiring vocabulary as "unanalyzed wholes" rather than having a rule-based phonological system, as seen in older children during the phonemic stage of acquisition. A broad-based assessment of toddlers' phonological skills would include age-appropriate words with a variety of sound classes and syllable/word structures that have a low phonetic complexity, which reflects typical speech and language development of young children.

In addition to the clinical purposes of a developmentally appropriate phonology test to determine if a child's phonology is developing as expected for early identification that can lead to early intervention, such a test would also be valuable for research purposes for comparing phonologies across children. To this end, we have developed an assessment that supports both clinicians and researchers who work with toddlers.

Acknowledgments

The publication of PEEPS™ has been similar to raising a child—there were ups and downs, delays, and years of work. We gave birth to the idea of PEEPS in 2006 and set to work identifying developmentally appropriate words based on age of acquisition and phonetic characteristics. Over the intervening years, we tested PEEPS on typically developing children ages 18–36 months in an iterative process: refining the word list, the elicitation procedures, and included additional age groups at 3-month intervals. We would like to thank the Directors of the East Tennessee State University Early Childhood Center and Little Bucs Laboratory Program for helping us recruit approximately 140 children whom we tested. We thank the children and their families for permitting us to test their children in the development of PEEPS. There have also been a number of graduate assistants who have helped with data collection and analysis over the years. We especially would like to acknowledge Morgan Johnson Geise, Grayson Evans Cathy, Kevanté Drew, and Javan Marshall, as well as Millie Newport Keathley, who photographed the sample toys shown in Chapter 3. We are also grateful for the clinicians who reviewed PEEPS and provided feedback on the forms and instructions. In particular, we thank Doanne Ward-Williams, Laura Vencill, and Marie Johnson, whose feedback improved the clarity and use of PEEPS.

Early supporters in the development of PEEPS included Sharynne McLeod from Charles Sturt University and Elise Baker from Western Sydney University, who provided feedback on words to make them appropriate for Australian/British/New Zealand English-speaking children. Both Sharynne and Elise have contributed to our thinking in the development of PEEPS.

We also would like to thank a number of researchers who have used PEEPS in their own research. Nancy Scherer and Ann Kaiser incorporated PEEPS in their intervention studies with young children who have cleft lip/palate; thanks to Rosemary Hodges and her dissertation committee (Elise Baker, Natalie Munro, and Karla McGregor), who used PEEPS in her study of LTs. In addition, we are grateful to our international colleagues who translated PEEPS into Swedish (Anette Lohmander, Anna Persson, Ulrika Marklund, and Fancisco Lacerda) and Brazilian Portuguese (Simone Nicolini de Simoni and Marcia Keske-Soares).

We want to thank everyone on the Brookes Publishing team who has patiently worked with us over the years. Special thanks to Astrid Zuckerman for not giving up and for passing us on to the very capable hands of Liz Gildea; Tess Hoffman, the most amazing editor we could ever imagine; and Ashley Wagner, Nicole Schmidl, and Savannah Neubert, who kept everything moving smoothly through all stages of production. The world of speech-language pathology is a better place thanks to the quality publications produced by the exceptional team at Paul H. Brookes Publishing.

We are grateful for the top-notch videos produced by Harold "Buddy" Arnold in the East Tennessee State University Broadcast Studio, along with Stacy Whitaker, Director of Engineering in the Department of Media and Communication. They are masterful in creating a clinical setting in a studio to produce professional video demonstrations that link the words in the Examiner's Manual to what it looks like to administer PEEPS to young, and often curious, children.

Finally, we thank our families, who have steadfastly supported us over the years of developing, testing, and writing PEEPS. To each of you we just want to say, we did it!

1 Introduction to PEEPS™

Profiles of Early Expressive Phonological Skills™ (*PEEPS*™) is a comprehensive test of early phonological skills in young children. It was designed to provide an easy, convenient, and developmentally appropriate way to examine the phonological skills of children 18–36 months of age in a detailed manner. The sections that follow provide a rationale for PEEPS and information on the background and development of the test.

RATIONALE: WHY DO WE NEED A PHONOLOGICAL TEST FOR TODDLERS?

Considerable attention has been given to the semantic and syntactic properties of early words, with the phonological properties being examined less often. There is evidence that phonology impacts early lexical development and the two interact during the early stages of acquisition (Sosa & Stoel-Gammon, 2012; Stokes, 2014; see also Stoel-Gammon, 2011 for a review of studies).

Lexical Selection

An example of this impact is *lexical selection*, in which a child's early vocabulary is selected in part based on the phonological characteristics of the words. That is, the phonological characteristics of selected words involve aspects of phonology that the child is capable of producing. There are several case studies that illustrate lexical selection in typically developing children. For example, Ferguson and Farwell (1975) reported a child's early vocabulary included words with sibilants (*cereal, shoes, juice, eyes, cheese, sit*). Stoel-Gammon and Cooper (1984) reported a child had several vocabulary words that ended in velars (*quack, rock, clock, sock, whack, milk, yuk, block, walk*). Lexical selection has also been observed in children with atypical development. In their article on phonological assessment in young children, Stoel-Gammon and Stone (1991) highlighted the lexical selection patterns evident in a 22-month-old child with a very limited productive vocabulary, only 15 words, 12 of which had labial consonants (*mama, balloon, book, ball, airplane, bye-bye, bottle, bus, apple, bath, peek-a-boo, bad boy*).

Schwartz and Leonard (1982) designed an experiment to test the idea of lexical selection. They developed a set of individualized nonsense words for each child in the study that included IN words that consisted of sounds that were IN the child's phonetic inventory and OUT words that included sounds that the child was not able to produce. They paired the nonsense words with an unusual toy or item and presented these to the children in a controlled number of presentations. When children were asked to name the items, they verbally named more IN words than OUT words, although there was no difference in comprehension (pointing to) the IN and OUT words. These findings support the concept of lexical selection and the impact of phonology on lexical acquisition.

Case studies of typical and atypical development in young children, along with experimental studies, provide evidence that individual children select words for their early vocabulary based in part on the phonological features of the words. Thus, selection of words is linked to a child's phonological abilities.

Lexical selection has also been examined using group data from the MacArthur Communicative Developmental Inventories (CDIs; Fenson et al., 1993; 2007; Marchman et al., 2023) that includes data from several thousand children acquiring English. Stoel-Gammon (1988) completed a phonetic analysis of the early acquired CDI words, which were words that 50% of the children produced at an early age. Her results also illustrate lexical selection in that the early acquired CDI words included stops, glides, and nasals (manner) as well as bilabials and alveolars (place), which matched the sounds of babble.

Collectively, these studies demonstrated the following links that exist in lexical-phonological development:

- Phonological abilities are linked to the selection of words for early vocabulary.

- Phonology of early words mirrors the phonetics of babble in terms of manner, place, and syllable shapes.

Phonological Development and Vocabulary Size

Another link between lexical and phonological development is that large vocabularies are associated with more advanced phonological systems. Likewise, smaller vocabularies are associated with less advanced phonological systems. The average lexicon size for a 24-month-old child with typical development is 250–300 words. This factor limits the range of words that can be included in a test of phonology. The phonological systems of Late Talkers (LTs; children with delayed vocabulary acquisition with fewer than 10 words at 18 months and fewer than 50 words at 24 months), compared with those of their age-matched peers, had fewer consonants in their phonetic inventory, less complex syllable structures, and lower accuracy of consonants. Their phonological systems resembled those of younger children. This provides additional support that lexical development and phonological development are commensurate and further illustrates the need for a developmentally appropriate test.

The clinical implication of these studies is that phonological development is more closely associated with vocabulary size than with age. This information is important for assessing the phonological systems of children with small vocabularies. As a consequence, phonological assessment of LTs and other children with limited vocabularies, including children with cleft palate, hearing impairment, autism, and cognitive delays, should not be based on traditional articulation tests. Rather, the best means of assessing the phonological skills of these children is by eliciting words that are likely to be in the vocabulary of young children with typical development. In addition to the clinical purposes of a developmentally appropriate phonology test to determine if a child's phonology is developing as expected for early identification that can lead to early intervention, such a test would also be valuable for research purposes for comparing phonologies across children.

Currently the available articulation/phonology tests are designed for a wide age range from toddlers to adults. Most contain vocabulary items that are unfamiliar to 2-year-olds, utilize elicitation techniques that are designed for children ages 3 years and older, and have brief administration times of 5–10 minutes. Of the 55 articulation and phonology tests listed in the American Speech-Language-Hearing Association (ASHA) Directory of Speech-Language Pathology Assessment Instruments (2007), only four indicate they can be used at 24 months. A description of the age range and administration time for these four tests in provided in Table 1.1.

Based on the large age range designated for currently available tests for assessing toddlers, these tests are not appropriate. A large proportion of words on a standard assessment test do not include the vocabulary of young children. The best means of assessing phonology in these

Table 1.1. Articulation and phonology tests that can be used at age 24 months

Test	Age Range	Administration Time
Arizona Articulation Phonology Scale-4 (Arizona-4) Fudala (2017)	18 months–22 years	5–20 minutes
Computerized Articulation and Phonology Evaluation System (CAPES) Masterson & Bernhardt (2001)	2 years–adult	Varies
Goldman-Fristoe Test of Articulation-3 (GFTA-3) Goldman and Fristoe (2015)	2–22 years	5–15 minutes
Hodson Assessment of Phonological Patterns-3 (HAPP-3) Hodson (2004)	2 years and up	15–20 minutes

children is by eliciting words that are likely to be in the vocabulary of young children with typical development. Consequently, there is a need for a developmentally appropriate test to assess the early phonological skills of children 18–36 months of age. PEEPS differs from traditional tests in that the primary factor for choosing test words is the likelihood that they will be part of the productive vocabulary of young children with typical development.

BACKGROUND AND DEVELOPMENT OF PEEPS

Given the well-documented evidence that the size of productive vocabulary and phonological development are linked in young children, the PEEPS Word List is specifically designed to include words that are likely to be familiar to young children and to those populations with limited expressive vocabularies. The following desirable features are included in this age-appropriate test for toddlers:

- Words that are present in the productive vocabularies of young children (18–24 months)

- Words with a variety of sound classes and syllable/word structures

- Methods of elicitation that encourage spontaneous productions and also allow for multiple prompts from the clinician or researcher

Stoel-Gammon and Williams (2013) noted that several sources of data are needed to obtain a comprehensive picture of a child's expressive phonology. Typically, for young children, that involves collecting a spontaneous speech sample. This sample will provide information on a child's "typical" productions with regard to lexicon, phonology, syntax, and pragmatics, along with a general idea of their speech intelligibility. However, this sample alone may not fully represent the child's phonological abilities because of lexical selection to produce words that are IN the child's phonetic inventory. Another limitation of spontaneous speech samples is the lack of comparability across samples, particularly for research purposes. To ensure a more representative sample, an articulation or phonological test is administered in addition to a spontaneous speech sample. In traditional tests, the test words are primarily monosyllabic and are selected based solely on their phonetic characteristics to elicit all consonants at least once in initial, medial, and final positions with some consonant clusters included. For example, the consonant /k/ might be tested in the words *cow, chicken,* and *book.* Some tests are designed to elicit specific phonological patterns, such as final consonant deletion, stopping, and fronting. Regardless of articulation or phonology tests, many of the test words are unfamiliar to young children, as noted previously. For example, several words from the Goldman-Fristoe Test of Articulation are acquired after age 4 (*lamp, drum, ring*) (Morrison et al., 1997). Given that the average lexicon size for a 24-month-old child with typical development is 250–300 words, the range of words that can be included in a test of phonology is limited. PEEPS differs from traditional articulation/phonology tests by including test words that are likely part of the productive vocabulary of young children, which is the primary factor for the word selection.

Once a representative and developmentally appropriate sample has been collected, independent and relational analyses must be completed to get a comprehensive picture of the phonological systems of 2-year-olds (Stoel-Gammon & Dunn, 1985). ***Independent analyses*** focus on the child's productions without comparison to the target words and provide information about the size and nature of the child's phonetic inventory in terms of place, voice, and manner of sounds produced, as well as the syllabic or word structure characteristics of their productions, such as complex structures including cluster production and multisyllabic words. ***Relational analyses*** are traditional ways that clinicians have described children's speech in terms of errors in relation to the adult target. Information is derived regarding accuracy, such as Percentage of Consonants Correct (PCC; Kwiatkowski & Shriberg, 1983) and error patterns, such as final consonant deletion and cluster reduction.

What Is the Population With Whom PEEPS Is Used?

PEEPS was developed for children 18–36 months of age or older who have small vocabularies and limited phonetic inventories. This would include LTs, children with cleft palate, children with hearing impairment, children diagnosed with autism, and children with cognitive delays. One such subset test by Scherer et al. (2012) used 10 words.

Who Initiates the Assessment Process?

The assessment process can be initiated by anyone who has a concern about a child's speech development. While it is often the parents/family who are the first to notice a delay, it is not uncommon for childcare providers, early childhood educators, or a pediatrician to bring the concern to the parents or request a referral for an evaluation by a speech-language pathologist. These professionals are often able to identify slower development in relation to other children in their care who are the same age.

Who Administers PEEPS?

Speech-language pathologists can administer PEEPS in a clinical setting. They have specialized training in phonetic transcription, knowledge of typical phonological and lexical acquisition, as well as clinical training on how to interact with and elicit a sample from a young child. PEEPS is not designed to be administered by anyone without this expertise. In the sections and chapters that follow, "speech-language pathologist" and "clinician" are used interchangeably to refer to the professional who administers PEEPS and interprets results.

How Long Does the Assessment Take?

The amount of time to administer PEEPS varies depending on several factors, including the age of the child, their attention to the task, as well as the size of their vocabulary. The average administration time ranged from 11 to 18 minutes across all ages. Typically developing 18-month-old children completed the test in the least amount of time (around 11 minutes) due to the smaller number of items they named (around 18 words), while 24-month-old children took the longest amount of time (around 22 minutes) and produced an average of 36 words. For children with cleft lip and palate, the administration time (around 11 minutes for 18-month-olds and 18 minutes for 24-month-olds) and number of words produced (17 and 29 words, respectively for 18- and 24-month-olds) were comparable to typically developing children of those ages (Scherer et al., 2012).

In addition to administering PEEPS, the clinician may want to collect a sample of the child's spontaneous speech. This will give the clinician an idea of the child's typical vocabulary, interaction in terms of initiations and responsiveness, and overall speech intelligibility. This would add an additional 15–20 minutes to PEEPS single-word elicitation.

Who Uses the Results and for What Purpose?

The clinician uses the results to make a determination of the child's phonological development. Information from PEEPS' independent and relational analyses guide the clinician in determining if the child is developing within expected limits, is delayed relative to age peers but displays a developmental sequence similar to typical development at a younger age, or displays "red flags" in unusual substitution and deletion errors, in addition to a smaller phonetic inventory and simpler syllable structure.

WHAT IS A PROFILE?

Within the PEEPS assessment protocol, the term *profile* refers to a multilayered description of a child's phonological system based on data from an assessment test designed specifically for young children. In the summary section of this guide, the term *profile* refers to expectations about the phonological system of typically developing children at 18, 24, 30, and 36 months (Chapter 6). The following description provides details on the profiles for individual children.

Individual Profiles

Analysis of the words produced by each child yields information regarding the *phonetic elements* of word productions including consonants, vowels, syllable and word structures, and stress patterns. They also describe the *accuracy* of productions.

Phonetic Elements   The phonetic measures in the PEEPS analyses include:

- A *list of consonants and consonant clusters* produced in word-initial and word-final positions

- The *number of different consonants/consonant clusters* produced in word-initial and word-final position

- The *phonetic features* (place and manner sound classes) of consonants produced in word-initial and word-final positions and the *number* of different place and manner classes in word-initial and word-final position

- A list of common word and syllable shapes occurring in the child's productions

These measures provide an inventory of the "building blocks" that the child uses in the formation of words; specifically, they identify the *consonants* and *consonant clusters* in the child's inventory and the word positions in which these elements occur.

The positional information included in the analyses is a critical part of the description as it specifies limits on use of the "building blocks" in particular word positions. For example, the inventory of a 21-month-old, Johnny, may show that he produces 8 different consonants in word-initial position, but none in word-final position; in contrast, the inventory of 24-month-old, Susie, may show that [b] and [d] are part of her consonantal repertoire only in word-initial but not word-final position, while [t] and [k] occur only in the end of words. Positional patterns such as these are an integral part of a child's profile.

In addition to these phonetic elements in a child's repertoire, the PEEPS analysis provides a *list of word and syllable structures* in the target words in terms of consonants (Cs) and vowels (Vs) and identifies which structures were produced by the child. The number of syllables that can occur in the word is also noted: that is, does the child produce two-syllable words? Does the child produce three-syllable words?

Finally, the profile may include additional comments that will be of interest in interpreting the findings. Examples of such comments include:

- Observations of the child's willingness to participate in the session (i.e., to produce the target words)

- The nature of "errors" in the child's productions (e.g., substitutions, assimilations, deletions, and vowel errors)

- Unusual error patterns in the child's productions (e.g., red flags)

Accuracy Measures   The *accuracy* measures in the PEEPS analyses are based on comparisons of the target word and the child's productions. These include the following:

- Accuracy (match) of initial and final consonant(s) for each word produced

- Accuracy (match) of word structures for each word produced

- Calculation of the total PCC for all words (and consonants in all positions) in the sample

In addition to the quantitative measures listed above, the profile includes the total number of words produced in the session and designates each word as spontaneous or imitated.

Interpretation and Clinical Applications of Individual Profiles

Individual profiles can be compared with profiles of typically developing children to determine if the child's phonological system is within normal limits. Identification of deficits in a child's profile can be used as a basis for developing an appropriate intervention program.

PHONOLOGICAL DEVELOPMENT IN TYPICALLY DEVELOPING CHILDREN

Acquisition of the sound system has been described in terms of four stages of development:

1. Prelinguistic Stage (birth to 1 year)

2. First Words Stage (1 year to 1 year, 6 months)

3. Phonemic Development Stage (1 year, 6 months to 4 years)

4. Stabilization of the Phonological System Stage (4 years to 8 years)

Prelinguistic Stage

Within the *Prelinguistic Stage*, the infant moves from reflexive vocalizations (such as crying, fussing, coughing, and burping) to nonreflexive vocalizations (including cooing, vocal play, and babbling). At the end of this stage, babbled utterances and the first meaningful words co-occur. That is, real words are embedded in babbled phrases.

First Words Stage

In the *First Words Stage*, there are two critical components in this stage of acquisition. First, the early words are learned and produced as *whole units* rather than as sequences of segments. That means that the child does not have a phonological rule that simplifies their production of the words. As a consequence, children at an early age can produce some words more accurately than they do at a later age. The "unanalyzed wholes" of word learning in this stage also result in variability in children's productions at this stage. For example, a child might produce the word "dog" variably as [dɑg], [dɑ], or [gɑg]. At this stage of development, there is not a stable correspondence between the child's productions and the adult targets as there is once the child moves to the rule-based stage of acquisition in the Phonemic Development Stage.

The second critical component of the First Words Stage is *active selection and avoidance*. An interesting aspect of the word learning that occurs in this stage involves the words that young children choose to include in their vocabularies (Ferguson & Farwell, 1975; Stoel-Gammon, 2011). It was once believed that children choose words based on the semantic and grammatical properties which allowed them to name objects or people, describe or demand an action, and interact socially with others. We now know that the phonological characteristics of the words play an important role in determining which words a child includes in their early vocabulary. Evidence from a number of studies indicates that children select and avoid words based on the phonological characteristics of those words. Specifically, children actively select words with phonological characteristics that are consistent with their developing sound systems and avoid words with characteristics that are outside their sound system. This strategy for vocabulary acquisition is evident in the first 50 words stage of language development and represents the very close intertwining of language and phonological skills at this age.

These two critical aspects of the First Words Stage (unanalyzed wholes and selectivity) have important implications for evaluating the phonological skills of young children and are the basis for the development of PEEPS as described below. Given that children actively use words that are consistent with their phonological skills, it is important to obtain an elicited sample that includes opportunities for the child to attempt words that are outside their phonology. If a language sample alone was the basis for examining a young child's phonology, it is likely that we would obtain a non-representative view of their abilities. Further, we need a sample that is sufficient to provide multiple exemplars of different phonetic characteristics across a number of words in order to check consistency and variability of children's early phonological skills.

Phonemic Development Stage

The *Phonemic Development Stage* signals the child's change from the whole-word approach to *rule-governed* forms that have a stable segmental correspondence with the adult words. This change occurs as a result of the rapid increase in vocabulary, which forces the child to move from the inefficient whole-word approach to a rule-based approach to vocabulary learning. The whole-word strategy was sufficient for the young child up to a 50-word vocabulary, but after that point, the child's rapid acquisition of vocabulary, up to 300 words by age 2, requires the child to develop a rule-based approach. The rule-based approach, then, results in the development of a sound system that is based primarily on phonemes rather than on whole words. In sum, two important characteristics of the Phonemic Development Stage are: 1) the rapid increase in vocabulary size and a relaxation of the selection constraints on adult words that the child attempts to produce; and 2) the relationship develops between the sounds of the adult words and the child's pronunciations, which becomes more stable and systematic.

Stabilization of the Phonological System Stage

Stabilization of the Phonological System is the final stage of phonological acquisition and represents the child's stabilization of consonants that had been variably produced, as well as acquisition of the last phonemes required for completion of their phonetic inventory. Developmental norms are frequently used to determine when those final consonants should be acquired. Refer to the section on *Speech Acquisition Norms* below.

EXPECTATIONS FOR THE
PHONOLOGICAL SYSTEM OF CHILDREN 18–36 MONTHS

At 18–24 months, the children whose phonological skills could be examined with PEEPS will likely be in the First Words Stage or the early Phonemic Development Stage. For these children, sitting at a table looking at pictures from a standardized sound inventory test would not be appropriate from a developmental standpoint. Using a broad-based analysis, PEEPS takes into account variability, active selection, and interest in books and interacting with toys that are characteristic of this age group.

Previous research shows that the phonological profiles of 2-year-olds with typical development are likely to show a limited set of consonant classes and word structures. Consonants occurring in word productions typically include voiced and voiceless stops, nasals, glides, some fricatives, and maybe a liquid. In terms of word structure, productions are likely to include V, CV, CVC, CVCV, CVCVC, and some clusters. Consonantal accuracy in running speech, measured by PCC, is about 70% at 24 months, and the proportion of speech that can be understood by a stranger (a measure of intelligibility) is about 50% (Stoel-Gammon, 1985; 1987).

The child's phonological system shows dramatic changes between 24 and 36 months with growth/improvement in all measures. According to Stoel-Gammon (1985, 1987) by 33–36 months, the inventory of consonants typically includes exemplars from all place and manner consonant classes. Word structures expand to include consonant clusters and words with 3–4 syllables. Consonantal accuracy in running speech, measured by PCC, is about 85%, and the proportion of speech that can be understood by a stranger (a measure of intelligibility) is around 75%.

For children's speech, the term *intelligibility* refers to the proportion of speech that can be understood by adults unfamiliar with the child. This measure varies with the context and, crucially, with the listener; most measures of intelligibility report the proportion of speech that can be understood by a "stranger" (i.e., an individual who is not familiar with the child's speech). The level of intelligibility increases when the listener is a parent or an individual familiar with the child's speech, and also when the context is known (e.g., when the child says [gɑ] while pointing to a dog). If a child's speech is difficult to understand, the problem may be associated with atypical phonological development, particularly with a limited set of consonants and restricted word shape patterns.

Speech Acquisition Norms

In a cross-linguistic review of children's acquisition of consonants in 27 languages, McLeod and Crowe (2018) summarized findings from over 60 studies from more than 30 countries on over 26,000 children to describe the overall patterns of speech sound development to aid clinicians in determining what is considered typical across languages. The outcome of their review showed that, across studies and across languages, most consonants are acquired by the age of 5 years. In a follow-up study, Crowe and McLeod (2020) completed a similar review of age of acquisition of consonants for children acquiring English in the United States. This second review involving U.S. children's speech acquisition involved 15 studies of almost 19,000 children. Similar to the findings of sound acquisition across 27 languages, Crowe and McLeod's results showed that most consonants were acquired by age 5.

The authors created a graphic for the acquisition of consonants to illustrate the average age across studies in which 90% of U.S. children produced specific sounds correctly (Crowe & McLeod, 2020). This chart is shown in Figure 1.1 and reproduced with permission. As shown in this graphic, children acquire most speech sounds by age 5;0.

Of particular interest is the acquisition of consonants by U.S. children at ages 2 and 3. As illustrated in the graph, at the 90% criterion level, all stops, nasals, and glides were acquired (i.e., produced correctly) on average by age 3;11. This corresponds with McIntosh and Dodd (2008), who reported that at the 90% criterion level, the phonetic repertoires (i.e., consonants produced, regardless of accuracy) of 2-year-olds included voiced and voiceless stops at all three places of articulation, nasals [m, n], glide [w], and fricative [s]. The remainder of the Crowe and McLeod chart shows that all affricates were acquired by age 4;11; all liquids acquired by 5;11, and the voiced interdental fricative [ð] is acquired by 6;11. The U.S. norm chart will be a valuable resource for U.S. clinicians.

There are three important points to share here: First, the results indicated that most consonants were reported to be acquired by the age of 5;0. This is younger than individual norm studies have reported or have been interpreted to show, which leads to the second point. That is, different norms use different methods of interpreting and displaying the data and therefore reading the norms the same way can lead to incorrect interpretations. Therefore, norms cannot be used to determine an age at which a child qualifies for therapy. Thirdly, norms should not be used in isolation for determining what is typical and what is atypical development. They provide one source of information which should be used with other information, such as stimulability and intelligibility (which includes examining whether the child produces typical or atypical error patterns).

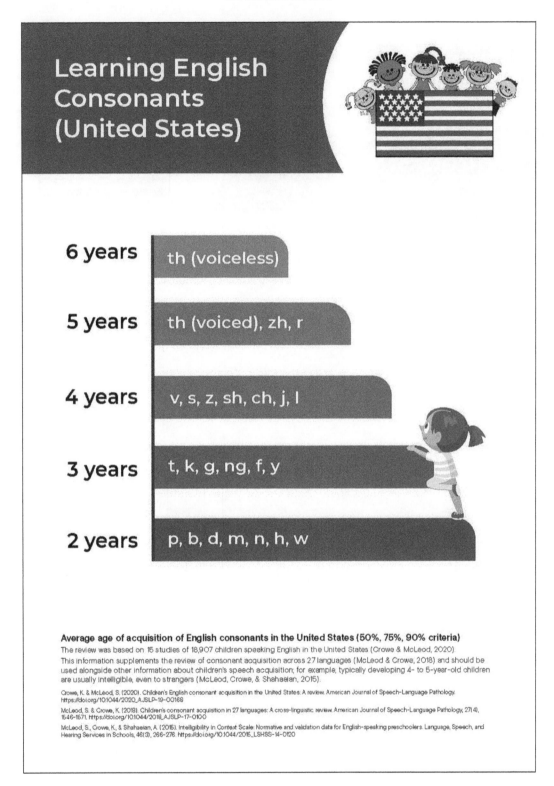

Figure 1.1. Average age of acquisition of English consonants in the United States, in a) bar graph representation and b) plot graph representation. (Reprinted by permission of Sharynne McLeod and Kathryn Crowe. Based on data from Crowe, K., & McLeod, S. [2020]. Children's English consonant acquisition in the United States: A review. *American Journal of Speech-Language Pathology.* http://doi.org/101044/2020_AJSLP-19-00188)

Figure 1.1. *(continued)*

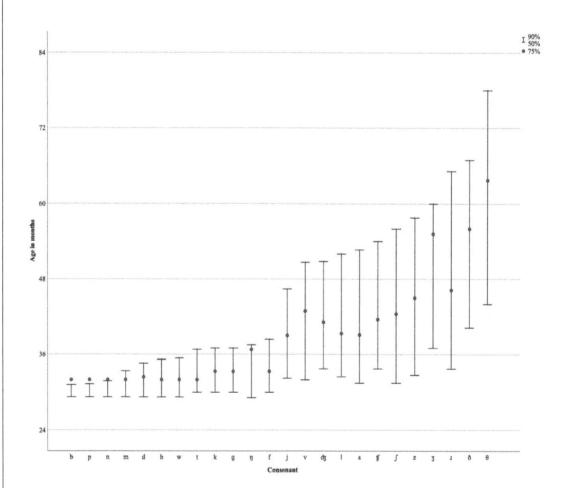

Average age of acquisition of English consonants in the United States (50%, 75%, 90% criteria)

The review was based on 15 studies of 18,907 children speaking English in the United States (Crowe & McLeod, 2020).

This information supplements the review of consonant acquisition across 27 languages (McLeod & Crowe, 2018) and should be used alongside other information about children's speech acquisition; for example, typically developing 4- to 5-year-old children are usually intelligible, even to strangers (McLeod, Crowe, & Shahaeian, 2015).

Crowe, K. & McLeod, S. (2020). Children's English consonant acquisition in the United States: A review. American Journal of Speech-Language Pathology. https://doi.org/10.1044/2020_AJSLP-19-00168

McLeod, S. & Crowe, K. (2018). Children's consonant acquisition in 27 languages: A cross-linguistic review. American Journal of Speech-Language Pathology, 27(4), 1546-1571. https://doi.org/10.1044/2018_AJSLP-17-0100

McLeod, S., Crowe, K., & Shahaeian, A. (2015). Intelligibility in Context Scale: Normative and validation data for English-speaking preschoolers. Language, Speech, and Hearing Services in Schools, 46(3), 266-276. https://doi.org/10.1044/2015_LSHSS-14-0120

Interactions Between Lexical and Phonological Development

As noted previously, it is well documented that the size of productive vocabulary and phonological development are linked in young children (see Stoel-Gammon, 2011 for a review of studies). In general, larger vocabularies are associated with larger phonetic inventories and more complex syllable and word structures. The PEEPS Word List is specifically designed to include words that are likely to be familiar to young children and to those populations with limited expressive vocabularies.

The age at which children produce their first word varies considerably. In some cases, parents report that their child said "dada" or "mama" at 8 months. The difficulty with pinpointing first word productions is that, although forms like [mɑmɑ], [pɑpɑ], or [dɑdɑ] are produced, these may be non-meaningful babbles rather than targeted words. When reinforced by parents, these forms often become real words. It is generally agreed that words other than "mama" or "dada" appear around 12–13 months and that by 15 months children have a productive vocabulary of about 10 words. Expressive vocabulary increases rapidly between 18 months and 24 months, rising from 50 words, on average, to 200–300 words over this 6-month period. Determining vocabulary size from 30 to 36 months is difficult, but research suggests that 30-month-old children produce about 450 words, and by 36 months vocabulary size has increased to 1,000 different words (Bowen, 2003).

The link between phonological and lexical development is apparent in studies of children who are slow in acquiring expressive vocabulary. In contrast to children with typical vocabulary acquisition, these children (again, often referred to as *Late Talkers*, or *LTs*), have fewer than 50 words in their expressive vocabulary at 24 months. Research shows that phonological development in this group is also slow, and is perhaps the cause of the delays in expressive vocabulary (Paul, 1993; Rescorla & Ratner, 1996; Stoel-Gammon, 1989; Williams & Elbert, 2003).

SUMMARY

Chapter 1 provided a rationale for a developmentally appropriate assessment for toddlers that is based on the important lexical-phonology link during that stage of development. Information on the development of PEEPS and a description of a profile were provided as the framework for the assessment followed by the description of the stages of phonological acquisition. Chapter 2 will build on this foundation with a detailed description of the components of the PEEPS Kit, including information on the words included to assess toddlers' phonological development and the PEEPS test forms, as well as guidelines on how to assemble the toys/objects for the kit.

PEEPS is a comprehensive test of early phonological skills in children ages 18–36 months. This chapter describes the components of the PEEPS Assessment Kit and the purpose of each component.

COMPONENTS INCLUDED IN THE PEEPS ASSESSMENT KIT

The PEEPS Assessment Kit includes the following components.

Examiner's Manual

The kit contains this manual with information on typical phonological development as well as information on PEEPS, the forms, administration, and interpretation of results.

Drawstring Bag for Storing Toys and Objects

To administer PEEPS, the examiner presents assorted toys and objects to the child, one by one, to elicit each corresponding word on the PEEPS Word List. A drawstring bag is included with the PEEPS Kit for storing these toys and objects. This allows for the examiner to have them all available for the PEEPS assessment and pull them out one at a time.

In most cases, the toys and objects are items clinicians are likely to have on hand or could easily obtain—e.g., a toy cow to represent the word *cow*; a baby doll to represent the words *baby* and *doll;* the doll's clothing and accessories to represent words such as *bottle, bib, diaper,* and *blanket.* Other words such as *hair* and *nose* can be elicited by pointing to body parts on oneself or the doll.

Board Book

Also included with the PEEPS test is a board book, *A Book of Things,* that includes illustrations of 12 words that the clinician may find difficult to represent with a toy or object at hand. These words are *banana, cheese, cookie, spoon, ball, balloon, soap, rock, zipper, train, watch,* and *block.*

Video Demonstrations

The PEEPS Demonstration Video, which is available for streaming (see the About the Video page at the front of this manual), shows PEEPS being administered to four children at ages 18 months, 23 months, 32 months, and 36 months. The video clips demonstrate the elicitation procedures using the cueing hierarchy described in Chapter 3 (spontaneous, cued, delayed imitation, and direct imitation), plus several other practices examiners will find helpful:

1. Recycling items to provide child with another attempt to name the item

2. Methods for eliciting words from different categories, including animals (names and sounds they make), body parts, food, clothing, and miscellaneous words (such as *balloon*)

3. Examples of redirecting behavior to the test items

The video includes brief text summaries to guide viewers' observations. For details about how to access this content, see the About the Video page at the beginning of this manual.

PEEPS Test Form

Finally, convenient record and analysis forms are included to summarize the data from the speech sample in order to analyze the following aspects of phonetic skills and phonological development:

- Phonetic inventory: Word-initial and word-final consonants occurring in the child's productions are listed by position and summarized by place and manner and classes

- Word structures in terms of consonants and vowels are compared with the structures of the target forms to determine if the structures match

- Proportion of word structures that match the target form

- Overall accuracy of consonant production using Percentage of Consonants Correct (PCC)

Information from these measures is compiled in the PEEPS test forms.

The PEEPS test form includes all of the information needed for the examiner to conduct *either* of two PEEPS assessments:

1. The full PEEPS assessment using the 60-word PEEPS Word List and corresponding Summary Analysis form, *or*

2. The PEEPS Screener, using a 20-word Screener Word List and corresponding Summary Analysis form.

The Screener will help clinicians determine if more in-depth testing using the full PEEPS assessment is warranted.

Thus, PEEPS includes two separate word lists: A 60-word list that includes lexical items that are acquired early in the speech of young children and a 20-word list that serves as a Screener. Each of these materials is described in the following sections.

Full PEEPS Word List and Summary Analysis   Target words in the PEEPS Word List were selected on the basis of two criteria: 1) the age of acquisition of each word and 2) the phonetic characteristics of the target words. The age of acquisition is based on an analysis of items from the MacArthur Communicative Development Inventories (CDIs) as noted in Fenson et al., 1993. *Age of acquisition* (AoA) was defined as the age at which at least *50% of children* produced the word according to parental report on the CDIs.

Target Words: Age of Acquisition   The PEEPS Word List includes 60 target words that occur in the expressive vocabulary of young children (see Appendix A at the back of this manual for AoA of all words). Using the criterion that acquisition occurs when at least 50% of the children have the word in their expressive vocabulary, all targets on the PEEPS Word List are "acquired" by 24 months according to the Stanford Wordbank website (http://wordbank.stanford.edu/). More specifically, 20 words are acquired by 18 months; 40 words by 21 months; and all 60 words by 24 months.

Target Words: Phonetic Characteristics In terms of phonetic characteristics, the target words include consonants in 7 places of articulation, 6 manner classes, and both voiced and voiceless consonants. Regarding word structures: 35 of the 60 words are early acquired word shapes: CV, CVC, or CVCV; four words have more than two syllables: *peek-a-boo, belly button, banana, elephant.* In addition, the words have few consonant clusters: 8 in word-initial position and 3 in word-final position.

The goal of the PEEPS assessment is to determine phonetic and phonological profiles of young children and those with limited expressive vocabularies. Thus, the PEEPS Word List differs from tests that assess all phonemes of English in initial and final (sometimes in initial, medial, and final) positions (see Stoel-Gammon & Williams, 2013). Target words in these tests vary considerably on AoA and phonetic complexity. In contrast to tests for older children, some late-acquired consonants do not occur in any target items on the PEEPS Word List, specifically [v, ð, ʒ], and others occur in few items, e.g., [θ].

The two developmental aspects of the vocabulary words (i.e., AoA and the phonetic characteristics of target words) are divided into "early" (18–21 months) and "later" (24–36 months) words. On the PEEPS test form, words typically acquired between the ages of 22 and 24 months are denoted with an asterisk. In this way, clinicians may choose to skip later words when administering PEEPS to children 18–21 months of age.

As shown in Figure 2.1, the PEEPS form for the full assessment provides detailed information on the consonants in the child's productions and on the word shapes that were produced. These elements, which can be considered the building blocks of phonological development, are fundamental to our analysis of the developing phonetic and phonological system. If the consonant inventories are smaller and/or if the word shapes are limited, word pronunciations will

INSTRUCTIONS

The *Profiles of Early Expressive Phonological Skills™*, or PEEPS™, is an instrument designed to measure expressive phonological skills in children ages 18–36 months. It is based on a set of 60 target words that typically developing children acquire by the age of 18–24 months. To conduct PEEPS, the examiner presents a stimulus to the child to elicit each target word, phonetically transcribes the child's production of each word, and then completes a phonetic and phonological analysis of the child's responses. It takes approximately 11–18 minutes to administer PEEPS and 10–20 minutes to summarize and analyze results. **Please refer to the PEEPS Examiner's Manual for detailed guidance on how to administer the test, record and analyze data, and interpret findings. See also the video demonstrations available with the PEEPS Assessment Kit.**

The examiner may conduct the full 60-word PEEPS assessment (pp. 2–5 of this form) or the 20-word Screener (pp. 6–7); to determine which to use, see the Manual. The essential steps of the testing process are the same for both. Either test may also be done remotely. See the Manual for guidance.

Prepare for Testing

1. Gather the stimuli used to elicit words: toys and the board book *A Book of Things.* Place toys in the drawstring bag, a foam cube, a pillowcase, or other container.
2. To create a naturalistic environment, test the child sitting on a blanket.
3. Plan to audio record the session so you can later check your transcriptions.

Elicit the Target Words and Transcribe Responses on the Word List

1. Present the container with toys (refer to the Manual for suggestions on how to organize the toys into semantic categories, i.e., animals, food, etc.). Allow the child to pull out only one toy at a time. (Similarly, focus on one stimulus at a time for the words that name body parts or that name objects shown in the board book.)
2. Excitedly ask, "What's that?"
3. Use the following cueing hierarchy to elicit the target word:
   • Spontaneous: "What is it?"
   • Cued: sentence completion, e.g., "On my foot, I wear a [*SHOE*]."
   • Delayed Imitation: forced choice with the target word given first, such as "Do you wear a SHOE or a spoon?"
   • Direct Imitation: "Say shoe."
4. Move through the cueing hierarchy at a reasonable pace.
5. Record data about the child's speech productions directly on the Word List. Target words are listed in column 1. The pre-completed cells to the right of each target word provide the target pronunciation (in IPA), word structure, initial consonant(s), final consonant(s), and total number of consonants. Use blank cells in these columns to transcribe data about the child's productions.

• *IPA: Child.* Enter a phonetic transcription of the child's production.
• *WSM.* Enter **1** if the child's production matches the target word structure form (e.g., CV). Enter **0** if it does not.
• *Initial C: Child.* Enter the initial consonant(s) of the child's production. For a deleted initial consonant, use a dash (-).
• *Final C: Child.* Enter the final consonant(s) of the child's production. For a deleted final consonant, use a dash (-).
• *S/I.* Label the child's production as spontaneous (**S**) or imitated (**I**). If more detail is desired, specify cued (**C**) or delayed imitation (**DI**).
• *PCC: Child.* Enter the number of consonants correct for the child's production. Remember to include medial consonants that occur in two- and three-syllable words.
• *Notes.* Enter any comments on the child's production, as needed.
• If the child does not respond to an item, enter **NR**. Enter **NT** if an item is not tested.
• See Manual instructions for tallying data for items that are marked **NR** or **NT** or items where the target pronunciation may vary, e.g., *kitty/cat).*

6. If a child produces fewer than 10 words, see the Manual for next steps.

Complete the Analysis Form

1. Complete the top section with information about the child, examiner name, test date, and total number of words the child produced.
2. Complete the Independent Analysis.
   • *Consonant Inventory.* Circle consonants and consonant clusters produced in each word position. Add consonants and clusters produced but not listed. Then fill in information for totals.
   • *Word and Syllable Shapes.* Circle those that occur.
   Number of syllables: 1 2 3
   Presence of: Final consonant(s) Initial consonant cluster
   Final consonant cluster
3. Complete the Relational Analysis.
   • *Accuracy—WSM.* Record the total WSM **# matches** from the bottom of column 5 on the Word List. Divide this by the total **# of words produced by child** to obtain a percentage score for WSM.
   • *Accuracy—PCC.* Record the PCC: **Child** total from the bottom of column 11 of the Word List. Divide this by the PCC: **Target** total at the bottom of column 12 to obtain a percentage score for PCC.
   • *Number of Syllables.* Circle Y/N to indicate if the child can produce 2- and 3-syllable words.
   • *Red Flags.* Circle Y/N to indicate if any red flags were noted; see the Manual for examples.

2

Figure 2.1. Pages from the PEEPS test form used for the full PEEPS assessment: a) instructions for examiner, b) Summary Analysis page, and c) 60-word Word List (20 words per page).

Figure 2.1. *(continued)*

PEEPS Summary Analysis and Word List

NOTES

Child's name:	Test age *(months)*:	# Words Produced:
Date of birth *(Y/M/D)*:	Gender:	
Date tested *(Y/M/D)*:	Examiner:	_____ / _____

Independent Analysis

Circle consonants and consonant clusters produced in each word position. Add consonants and clusters produced but not listed.

Consonant Inventory																			
Word-Initial Consonants	p	b	t	d	k	g	f	s	z	ʃ	tʃ	dʒ	m	n	l	ɹ	w	h	Other: / Total:
Word-Initial Clusters	bl-	tɹ-	dɹ-	kw-	sp-	st-													Other: / Total:
Word-Initial Manner	Stop		Fricative		Affricate		Nasal		Liquid		Glide		# Manner Classes:						
Word-Initial Place	Labial/labiodental		Alveolar/interdental		Palatal		Velar		Glottal		# Places:								
Word-Final Consonants	p	b	t	d	k	g	θ	f	s	z	ʃ	tʃ	m	n	ŋ	l	ɹ		Other: / Total:
Word-Final Clusters	-nd	-nt	-ŋk																Other: / Total:
Word-Final Manner	Stop		Fricative		Affricate		Nasal		Liquid		# Manner Classes:								
Word-Final Place	Labial/labiodental		Alveolar/interdental		Palatal		Velar		# Places:										

Word and Syllable Shapes: Circle those that occur.   **Number of syllables:** 1   2   3
Presence of: Final consonant(s)   Initial consonant cluster   Final consonant cluster

Relational Analysis

Accuracy		
# WS Match / # Words Produced: _____/_____	WSM: _____%
PCC Child / PCC Target: _____/_____	PCC: _____%

Number of Syllables	
2-syllable	Y / N
3-syllable	Y / N

Red Flags (See Manual for examples.)	
WF inventory substantially > WI inventory	Y / N
Unusual Vowel Errors	Y / N
Atypical Consonant Substitutions	Y / N
Atypical Deletions	Y / N

3

Word	IPA: Target	IPA: Child	WS Target	WSM	Initial C: Target	Initial C: Child	Final C: Target	Final C: Child	S/I	PCC: Child	PCC: Target	Notes
cow	kaʊ		CV		k						1	
moo	mu		CV		m						1	
dog	dɑg		CVC		d		g				2	
woof	wʊf		CVC		w		f				2	
duck(y)	dʌk(i)		CVC(V)		d		(k)				2	
quack	kwæk		CCVC		kw		k				3	
fish(y)	fɪʃ(i)		CVC(V)		f		(ʃ)				2	
bird	bɚd		CVC		b		d				2	
kitty (cat)	kɪt/di (kæt)		CVCV(CVC)		k		(t)				2 (4)	
puppy	pʌpi		CVCV		p						2	
*mouse	maʊs		CVC		m		s				2	
pig(gy)	pɪg(i)		CVC(V)		p		(g)				2	
*sheep	ʃip		CVC		ʃ		p				2	
chicken	tʃɪkən		CVCVC		tʃ		n				3	
bug	bʌg		CVC		b		g				2	
*elephant	ɛləfənt		VCVCVCC				nt				4	
*monkey	mʌŋki		CVCCV		m						3	
*lion	laɪ(j)ən		CV(C)VC		l		n				2 (3)	
baby	beɪbi		CVCV		b						2	
ear	ɪɹ		VC				ɹ				1	
# words produced by child/# words possible		# match							Total PCC			

*indicates words acquired between 22–24 months

4

Figure 2.1. *(continued)*

Word	IPA: Target	IPA: Child	WS Target	WSM	Initial C: Target	Initial C: Child	Final C: Target	Final C: Child	S/I	PCC: Child	PCC: Target	Notes
finger	fɪŋgɚ		CVCCV		f						3	
*foot	fʊt		CVC		f		t				2	
hair	hɛɹ		CVC		h		ɹ				2	
hand	hænd		CVCC		h		nd				3	
mouth	maʊθ		CVC		m		θ				2	
nose	noʊz		CVC		n		z				2	
toe(s)	toʊ(z)		CV(C)		t		(z)				1 (2)	
*tummy	tʌmi		CVCV		t						2	
*tongue	tʌŋ		CVC		t		ŋ				2	
belly button	bɛlibʌtən		CVCVCVCVC		b		n				5	
*soap	soʊp		CVC		s		p				2	
*comb	koʊm		CVC		k		m				2	
blanket	blæŋkət		CCVCCVC		bl		t				5	
peek-a-boo	pikəbu		CVCVCV		p						3	
*doll	dɑl		CVC		d		l				2	
shoe	ʃu		CV		ʃ						1	
*sock	sɑk		CVC		s		k				2	
*zipper	zɪpɚ		CVCV		z						2	
hat	hæt		CVC		h		t				2	
off	ɑf		VC				f				1	
# words produced by child/# words possible			# match						Total PCC			

*Indicates words acquired between 22–24 months

Word	IPA: Target	IPA: Child	WS Target	WSM	Initial C: Target	Initial C: Child	Final C: Target	Final C: Child	S/I	PCC: Child	PCC: Target	Notes
diaper	daɪpɚ		CVCV		d						2	
*bib	bɪb		CVC		b		b				2	
juice	dʒus		CVC		dʒ		s				2	
banana	bənænə		CVCVCV		b						3	
cookie	kʊki		CVCV		k						2	
cheese	tʃiz		CVC		tʃ		z				2	
cup	kʌp		CVC		k		p				2	
drink	dɹɪŋk		CCVCC		dɹ		ŋk				4	
bottle	bɑt/dəl		CVCVC		b		l				3	
spoon	spun		CCVC		sp		n				3	
*train	tɹeɪn		CCVC		tɹ		n				3	
truck	tɹʌk		CCVC		tɹ		k				3	
*stop	stɑp		CCVC		st		p				3	
go	goʊ		CV		g						1	
light	laɪt		CVC		l		t				2	
balloon	bəlun		CVCVC		b		n				3	
ball	bɑl		CVC		b		l				2	
*rock	ɹɑk		CVC		ɹ		k				2	
*block	blɑk		CCVC		bl		k				3	
*watch	wɑtʃ		CVC		w		tʃ				2	
# words produced by child/# words possible			# match						Total PCC			

*Indicates words acquired between 22–24 months

be affected. In some cases, the PEEPS analyses may show that the size of a child's inventory is within normal range, but the accuracy of word production, as assessed by relational measures, is low. In such cases, the problem may be associated with difficulties in using the phonetic inventory to achieve a match between the child's form and the adult target.

Target Words: Other Considerations In addition to the AoA and phonetic criteria, words were chosen that have international familiarity. In the few instances where there are differences in word labels between the American labels and their referents in other English-speaking countries, alternative labels are indicated. For example, the American words *diaper, cookie, cracker, kitty,* and *bug* could be elicited as the British, Australian, or New Zealand English equivalents of *nappy, biscuit, biscuit, cat,* and *bug/beetle,* respectively. Before adopting the target form into the word list, the AoA and phonetic characteristics of the target should be considered. Finally, multiple exemplars of the different phonetic characteristics were included across a number of words in order to check consistency and variability of children's early phonological skills.

PEEPS Screener Word List and Summary Analysis The PEEPS Screener, shown in Figure 2.2, contains 20 words from the 60-word list. As noted above, the purpose of the screener is to help clinicians determine if more in-depth testing using the full PEEPS is warranted. The Screener provides a convenient and efficient way to elicit words that sample all place, voice, and manner categories of English consonant production, as well as a variety of syllable structures across both early and later developing words. Analysis of words from the PEEPS Screener is the same as for the PEEPS Word List. A full description of the analyses is provided in Chapter 3.

Screener Summary Analysis and Word List

peeps

Child's name:	Test age *(months)*:	**# Words Produced:** ____ / ____	NOTES
Date of birth *(Y/M/D)*:	Gender:		
Date tested *(Y/M/D)*:	Examiner:		

Independent Analysis

Circle consonants and consonant clusters produced in each word position. Add consonants and clusters produced but not listed.

Consonant Inventory																				
Word-Initial Consonants	p	b	t	k		f	s	ʃ	dʒ	m	n	l	w	h					**Other:**	**Total:**
Word-Initial Clusters	tɹ-	dɹ-																	**Other:**	**Total:**
Word-Initial Manner	*Stop*			*Fricative*			*Affricate*			*Nasal*			*Liquid*			*Glide*			**# Manner Classes:**	
Word-Initial Place	*Labial/labiodental*					*Alveolar/interdental*				*Palatal*			*Velar*			*Glottal*			**# Places:**	
Word-Final Consonants	p	t	k	g	θ	s	z	tʃ	m	l									**Other:**	**Total:**
Word-Final Clusters	-nt	-ŋk																	**Other:**	**Total:**
Word-Final Manner	*Stop*					*Fricative*				*Affricate*			*Nasal*			*Liquid*			**# Manner Classes:**	
Word-Final Place	*Labial/labiodental*					*Alveolar/interdental*				*Palatal*					*Velar*				**# Places:**	

Word and Syllable Shapes: Circle those that occur. **Number of syllables:** 1 2 3

Presence of: Final consonant(s) Initial consonant cluster Final consonant cluster

Relational Analysis

Accuracy	
# WS Match / # Words Produced: ____/____	**WSM:** ____%
PCC Child / PCC Target: ____/____	**PCC:** ____%

Number of Syllables	
2-syllable	*Y / N*
3-syllable	*Y / N*

Red Flags (See Manual for examples.)	
WF inventory substantially > WI inventory	Y / N
Unusual Vowel Errors	Y / N
Atypical Consonant Substitutions	Y / N
Atypical Deletions	Y / N

Profiles of Early Expressive Phonological Skills™ (PEEPS™) by A. Lynn Williams and Carol Stoel-Gammon.

7

Figure 2.2. Pages used only for the PEEPS Screener assessment: a) Summary Analysis page, and b) 20-word Word List.

Figure 2.2. *(continued)*

Word	IPA: Target	IPA: Child	WS Target	WSM	Initial C: Target	Initial C: Child	Final C: Target	Final C: Child	S/I	PCC: Child	PCC: Target	Notes
dog	dɑg		CVC		d		g				2	
puppy	pʌpi		CVCV		p						2	
elephant	ɛlafant		VCVCVCC				nt				4	
baby	beɪbi		CVCV		b						2	
foot	fʊt		CVC		f		t				2	
mouth	maʊθ		CVC		m		θ				2	
nose	noʊz		CVC		n		z				2	
toe(s)	toʊ(z)		CV(C)		t		(z)				1 (2)	
comb	koʊm		CVC		k		m				2	
shoe	ʃu		CV		ʃ						1	
sock	sɑk		CVC		s		k				2	
hat	hæt		CVC		h		t				2	
juice	dʒus		CVC		dʒ		s				2	
banana	banænə		CVCVCV		b						3	
cup	kʌp		CVC		k		p				2	
drink	dɹɪŋk		CCVCC		dɹ		ŋk				4	
truck	tɹʌk		CCVC		tɹ		k				3	
light	laɪt		CVC		l		t				2	
ball	bɑl		CVC		b		l				2	
watch	wɑtʃ		CVC		w		tʃ				2	
# words produced by child/# words possible			# match						Total PCC			

8

OTHER ITEMS NEEDED TO ADMINISTER PEEPS

As noted above, the assessment procedure is the same whether the examiner is administering the PEEPS Screener or the full PEEPS assessment. The examiner presents a stimulus to the child to elicit the child's production of the target word. This stimulus may be 1) an object or toy pulled from a container, 2) a body part or article of clothing that the examiner points to, or 3) a picture in the board book *A Book of Things*.

The words on both the full PEEPS Word List and the Screener Word List name familiar items or concepts (e.g., *cow* and *moo*). Clinicians who work with young children will likely have many of these items on hand in their setting—toy animals, dolls, and the like. Others can be easily obtained. Chapter 3 provides detailed guidance for selecting and purchasing items needed to create a PEEPS toy collection.

SUMMARY

Chapter 2 described the PEEPS Kit, including the toys/objects, words, and test forms. In Chapter 3, information will be provided that describes how to assemble a toy test kit and then administer and analyze the data collected for PEEPS.

3 Administering PEEPS and Completing the Analysis

With Nancy J. Scherer

This chapter will provide guidelines and tips in preparing to administer PEEPS and in the procedures used to elicit a child's responses to PEEPS items. A step-by-step guide is provided in using the PEEPS forms to complete an independent and relational analysis. Finally, the chapter discusses additional clinical considerations for using PEEPS.

PREPARING TO ADMINISTER PEEPS

Of the 60-item PEEPS Word List, 12 words are illustrated in the board book *A Book of Things*. The remaining 48 words are represented by toys. Note that one toy can be used to elicit more than one word. For example, a toy cow is used for the words *cow* and *moo*. Also, there are 10 body part words that can be elicited by pointing to those parts on the child, clinician, or baby doll. The annotated PEEPS Word List (in Appendix 3.1) shows which words are represented by toys, actions (e.g., stop/go; on/off), body parts, or illustrated in *A Book of Things*.

Note: *A Book of Things* is included in the PEEPS Kit so that the examiner can easily represent words naming certain items they might not have readily available, such as *banana*, *rock*, *cheese*, or a *watch*. However, if the examiner does have any of these items on hand, they may choose to use the physical object, rather than the picture in *A Book of Things*, to elicit the word. See the guidelines below for selecting physical objects and toys to include in a PEEPS toy collection.

Assembling the Objects/Toys

The PEEPS Word List in Appendix 3.1 provides a useful categorization of the 60 words into semantic categories, which will guide the clinician in assembling a PEEPS toy collection. These items can be purchased at retail stores or online. Most of the PEEPS words can be grouped in the following semantic categories, which can guide your shopping for the toys.

Baby/Body Parts   This category contains 22 words that can be represented using toys.

- A baby doll with clothing items can be used to elicit the words *baby, doll, sock, shoe, hat, bib,* and *diaper* and can include baby items for *blanket, peek-a-boo, bottle,* and *comb.*

- Body parts represent 11 of the 22 words, which can be elicited by pointing to those parts on the child, clinician, or doll: *ear, finger, foot, tummy, hand, mouth, nose, toe, belly button, tongue,* and *hair.*

Animals   This category contains 18 words that can be represented using toys. (Note that a toy may represent multiple words. For example, the same toy might be used for *duck* and *quack*.)

- Farm animals (or animal sounds): *bird, cow, moo, mouse, kitty, duck, quack, dog, puppy, woof, pig, chicken, bug, sheep.*

- Jungle animals: *lion, elephant, monkey.*

- Other: *fish.*

Food   This category contains 7 words that can be represented using 1 toy and 4 illustrations in *A Book of Things*.

- A toy cup can be used to elicit the words *juice, cup, drink.*

- The food words *banana, cheese, cookie,* and *spoon* are illustrated in the board book.

Miscellaneous   This category contains 13 words that can be represented using 2 toys and 8 illustrations in *A Book of Things*.

- A toy truck can be used to elicit the words *truck, go,* and *stop.*

- A flashlight can be used to elicit the words *light* and *off.*

- The words *ball, balloon, soap, rock, zipper, train, watch,* and *block* are illustrated in the board book.

Tips: Dos and Don'ts for Selecting Toys   As you gather toys for your PEEPS collection, there are two very important considerations. First, toys should be large enough—at least 1¼ inches (3 centimeters) in diameter and 2¼ inches (6 centimeters) in length to avoid being swallowed or lodged in the child's throat. You can use a small-parts tester, or choke tube, to determine if a toy is too small. A rule of thumb is to choose toys larger than a child's mouth. Choose plastic toys that are sturdy and have a label that says "nontoxic."

Secondly, choose plastic or washable toys, rather than cloth toys, so that you can easily clean them after each test session. It is recommended that you soak the toys in a sink with a half-cup of bleach per gallon of water. Allow the toys to soak for 5 minutes, rinse, and air dry before using them again.

A final tip: do not select toys that make noise that will distract children and decrease their attention to the naming task. Avoid squeaky toys, musical toys, or toys with batteries.

Sample photos of the toys that can be collected to represent the PEEPS words are included in Appendix 3.2.

Setting Up the Environment

You will notice in the video demonstrations that the children were tested sitting on a blanket on the floor. For toddlers, sitting on the floor creates a more naturalistic environment than sitting in a chair at a table. The blanket also defines the space and focus for the child and clinician during the testing. In the video, the clinician can see the examiner redirect the child to sit on the blanket with them.

Designate a floor space to use while administering PEEPS. Make sure this area is free of clutter and distractions. Spread a blanket out in advance to define the space and make it comfortable and inviting.

Finally, it is strongly recommended you plan to audio record the testing session. Although the PEEPS form is set up to allow for transcribing data about the child's speech productions during testing, an audio recording allows you to check for accuracy.

Using the Test Form: Overview

The PEEPS test form includes material for administering the full PEEPS or the PEEPS Screener.

The first page of the test form provides an overview of testing procedures intended for the examiner's quick reference. These procedures are the same for both the full PEEPS and the Screener. For either, you will

1. Transcribe data about the child's word productions directly on the Word List during the testing session and/or afterward, along with any notes.

2. Use the bottom row of the Word List to begin summarizing and analyzing the data (e.g., tallying total number of words the child produced).

3. Use the Summary Analysis form to record basic information about the child and testing session, along with independent and relational analyses of the child's word productions.

Full PEEPS Assessment   If you are conducting the full PEEPS assessment, you will use pages 2–5 of the test form. Page 2 is used to provide information about the child, the date of testing, the examiner, the number of target words produced, and a summary of *independent* and *relational* analyses. It also includes a section in which the examiner or analyzer can add comments about the test session. Pages 3–5 provide the 60-word Word List, along with space for recording data about the child's word productions.

The child's productions are phonetically transcribed and then analyzed for phonetic and phonological properties. Although it is recommended that the sample be audio recorded for accuracy of recorded responses, the PEEPS form makes it possible for clinicians to complete online transcriptions of the child's production during the testing session; that is, transcribing while administering the test.

PEEPS Screener   There may be circumstances in which time is limited to conduct a full PEEPS assessment or the clinician wants to get a quick overview of a child's development without a detailed assessment of their phonological development. For these instances, the PEEPS Screener would be appropriate.

If you are conducting the PEEPS Screener, you will use pages 6–7 of the test form. Page 6 is used to provide basic information about the child and a summary of independent and relational analyses. Page 7 provides the 20-word Word List used for the screener, along with space for recording data about the child's word productions.

OBTAINING A SAMPLE AND TRANSCRIBING DATA

The PEEPS test is based on single-word responses to a set of stimuli. The video included with your PEEPS Kit demonstrates the test items and examples of elicitation techniques with four different children ranging in age from 18 to 36 months. The sections below describe the target words and provide suggestions for obtaining a sample.

Organizing Stimuli

Stimuli should be presented to the child one at a time. A drawstring bag is included with your PEEPS Kit. You can place a small number of the toys in the bag so that the child can put their hand in to pull out a toy to name. A pillowcase or a soft, machine-washable cube can be used for the same purpose. (In the photos of the toys and the video demonstrations, you will notice the latter option; the cube we used during development of PEEPS is available through Lakeshore Learning or other providers of teacher supplies.)

Before you begin, here is a tip to organize your toys for a convenient and easy way to work with the child to name the items. Separate the toys into the four semantic categories listed above using plastic storage bags. You can then place one of these bags into the drawstring bag provided with your PEEPS Kit (or a soft cube or pillowcase) for the child to pull them out one at a time. Once the child has pulled out each toy within a category, place them all back in the plastic storage bag, and pull out the next storage bag to put into the cloth bag or cube for the child to pull out. This organization will eliminate, or certainly reduce, potential chaos with too many toys in view to distract the child. It also will help keep the child's attention as new toys are hidden in the drawstring bag or cube. Once the child has named the items in a bag, the clinician can put the items away in the same bag, put the bag behind their back, and move to the next bag. This will help keep the child from being distracted by the toys that have already been named.

Remember, for some words, you will use an illustration in the board book *A Book of Things* to elicit the word, or you will point to a body part. Plan ahead for how you will elicit each word on the Word List you are using, so you can move through the list quickly during testing.

Eliciting the Child's Responses

To administer PEEPS, you will use the Word List to record information about the child's production of each word as you elicit words. The order in which the words are elicited does not matter, although it is generally easier for children to ease into the testing session if you begin with the animals, often followed by the baby items and body parts, food, and then miscellaneous toys. Allow the child to pull out only one toy at a time, and then excitedly ask "What's that?" The following cueing hierarchy can be used to elicit the word:

1. Spontaneous: "What is it?"

2. Cued: sentence completion, such as "You turn the flashlight on and [*OFF*]."

3. Delayed Imitation: forced choice with the target word given first, such as "Do you turn the flashlight OFF or swim?"

4. Direct Imitation: "Say *flashlight*."

It is recommended that you move through the cueing hierarchy at a reasonable pace so the child does not lose interest. This cueing hierarchy provides additional methods to elicit the words spontaneously. If you notice a consistent pattern in the child's responding, you may determine it is not productive to go through the entire cueing hierarchy in naming each toy. For some children, particularly at the younger ages, you may find that you move directly to Direct Imitation after Spontaneous. If the child still does not say the word, place the toy behind your back and pull it out again after you have gone through the items to see if the item is named with a second attempt.

The video demonstrates elicitation of the PEEPS words using the cueing hierarchy. Also, please note that the PEEPS Word List includes a column to record whether the child's response was spontaneous (S) or imitative (I). The same column appears on the Screener Word List. You will also record there if there was no response (NR), or the word was not tested (NT).

Transcribing the Responses

As you administer PEEPS, you may choose to record data about the child's speech productions directly on the Word List. Target words are listed in column 1. The pre-completed cells to the right of each target word provide the target pronunciation (in International Phonetic Alphabet, or IPA), word structure, initial consonant(s), final consonant(s), and total number of consonants. You will use the blank cells in these columns to transcribe data about the child's productions:

• *IPA: Child.* Enter a phonetic transcription of the child's production.

• *WSM.* Enter **1** if the child's production matches the target word structure form (e.g., CV). Enter **0** if it does not.

• *Initial C: Child.* Enter the initial consonant(s) of the child's production.

• *Final C: Child.* Enter the final consonant(s) of the child's production.

- *S/I.* Label the child's production as spontaneous **(S)** or imitated **(I).** If more detail is desired, specify cued **(C)** or delayed imitation **(DI).**

- *PCC: Child.* Enter the number of consonants correct for the child's production. Remember to include medial consonants that occur in two- and three-syllable words.

- *Notes.* Enter any comments on the child's production, as needed.

- If the child does not respond to an item, enter **NR.** Enter **NT** if an item is not tested.

The sections below describe in greater detail how to transcribe data for each column on the Word List as you conduct the assessment.

A broad transcription of the target word is provided as part of the assessment form and transcription of the child's productions can also be broad; attention should be given to the features of *place* and *manner* of consonants. Vowels in target words are provided in the assessment forms, using phonetic transcription of vowels of *General American English* (GAE). Within the United States, there is greater dialectal variation in the phonetic features of vowels than in consonants, and much greater variation in the pronunciation of vowels in other of the English-speaking regions of the world, with notable differences in the vowel production in the UK and Australia. Because the focus of the PEEPS analysis is on consonants, it is not necessary to identify minor differences between the vowel in the transcriptions of target words unless there is a major change in the vowel height (e.g., if the target [i] is produced as [o]) or in the front-back/rounding dimension (e.g., the target [ɪ] is produced as [o]). As shown in the analyses below, the focus of the PEEPS analysis is on the phonetic features and accuracy of consonants.

COMPLETING YOUR ANALYSIS ON THE TEST FORM

A detailed description of how to record data directly on the Word List is presented below, followed by explanation of how to complete the Summary Analysis page with summaries of the independent and relational analyses.

The last two lines of these pages show the number of words produced by the child, the number of Word Structure Matches (WSM), and the Percentage of Consonants Correct (PCC) counts for the child's productions and the target forms. Information from these lines is transferred to the overall summaries on page 1 (see below). The Summary Analysis page of the form includes information on the range of syllable structures in the child productions and any "red flags" that are noted in the "Notes" column. For ease of description, the examples below include headers that are identified with column numbers; these numbers do not appear on the actual PEEPS form. (See Appendices 3.3 and 3.4 at the end of this chapter, as well as the appendices to Chapter 5, for examples of completed forms.)

Data Entry Using the Word List

The PEEPS Word List has 60 words, 30 on each page, and the Screener Word List has 20 words. Descriptions of each of the columns on the PEEPS and Screener Word Lists are provided in the sections below.

Pre-entered Data   As shown in Figure 3.1, columns 1, 2, 4, 6, 8, and 12 contain pre-entered data, as follows.

Column 1   **Word** shows the target words in each of the assessment word lists. You may find when you elicit a particular target word, the child's production differs from the word appearing in column 1. For example, the target *kitty* may be produced as *cat* or *kitty cat.* In such cases,

1. The pre-entered data for the target word should be changed to reflect the child's form.

2. The IPA Target (Column 2), WS Target (Column 4), Initial C: Target and Final C: Target (Columns 6 and 8), and PCC Target (Column 11) must also be changed, if needed.

COL. 1	2	3	4	5	6	7	8	9	10	11	12	13
Word	IPA: Target	IPA: Child	WS Target	WSM	Initial C: Target	Initial C: Child	Final C: Target	Final C: Child	S/I	PCC: Child	PCC: Target	Notes
cow	kaʊ		CV		k						1	
moo	mu		CV		m						1	
dog	dag		CVC		d		g				2	
woof	wʊf		CVC		w		f				2	
finger	fɪŋgɚ		CVCCV		f						3	
banana	bənænə		CVCVCV		b						3	
fish(y)	fɪʃ(i)		CVC(V)		f		(ʃ)				2	
kitty (cat)	kɪt/di (kæt)		CVCV(CVC)		k		(t)				2(4)	
puppy	pʌpi		CVCV		p		p				2	
sheep	ʃip		CVC		ʃ		p				2	
chicken	tʃɪkən		CVCVC		tʃ		n				3	
bug	bʌg		CVC		b		g				2	
elephant	ɛləfənt		VCVCVCC				nt				4	
monkey	mʌŋki		CVCCV		m						3	
lion	laɪ(j)ən		CV(C)VC		l		n				2	
foot	fʊt		CVC		f		t				2	
cheese	tʃiz		CVC		tʃ		z				2	
hair	hɛɹ		CVC		h		ɹ				2	
hand	hænd		CVCC		h		nd				3	
mouth	maʊθ		CVC		m		θ				2	

Figure 3.1. Pre-entered data for 20 words.

Column 2   IPA Target provides a broad transcription of the target words. It should be noted that the vowels of target words may vary from one region to another (or one English-speaking country to another). Given that the PEEPS analyses focus primarily on consonants and word structures, precise transcription of vowels is not necessary. Unusual vowel productions can be noted in Column 13 (Notes) and may be considered "red flags." Two points are worth noting with regard to the IPA Target transcriptions:

1. You will notice the current IPA transcription for "r" is now written as /ɹ/.

2. The final "r" in the targets *ear* (IPA /ɪɹ/) and *hair* (IPA /hɛɹ/) is counted as a word-final consonant and appears in the list of final consonants as part of the phonetic inventory. In contrast, the /ɚ/ (as in *finger* and *zipper*) is counted as a rhotic vowel.

Column 4   WS Target shows the word structure of the target in terms of consonants (C) and vowels (V). As noted above, the CV structure is based on the target word produced by the child and should be modified as needed. For example, if the child's form is *doggy* rather than *dog*, the structure is CVCV rather than CVC.

Column 6   Initial C: Target shows the initial consonant(s) of the child's target word.

Column 8   Final C: Target shows the final consonant(s) of the target word. Note that if the child says fishy rather than fish, or *ducky* rather than *duck*, there is no final consonant on the target.

Column 12   PCC: Target shows the number of consonants in the target word.

Column 13   Notes allows you to enter comments regarding the production.
Figure 3.1 provides an example of pre-entered data for 20 words.

Data Entry for Child Productions: Columns 3, 5, 7, 9, 10, 11   For each target word, you will enter data as follows:

Column 3: IPA: Child   A phonetic transcription of the child's production is entered here. It is best to work from a recording of the test session although it is possible to transcribe online (i.e., while administering the test). (*Note:* A broad transcription is used for the IPA Target [Column 2] and is sufficient for the transcription of the child's production and the analyses to be performed.)

Column 5: WSM   WSM is a comparison of the CV structure of the target form and the child's production. This is a binary decision: Enter a "1" if the forms match or a "0" if they do not match. Remember that the WSM is based on the child's production: if the target is *kitty cat* and the child says *cat*, the Word Structure for Target is CVC and you will enter 1 in Column 5.

Column 7: Initial C: Child   The initial consonant(s) of the child's production is/are entered.

Column 9: Final C: Child   The final consonant(s) of the child's production is/are entered. *Note:* Use a dash (–) or other consistent mark to indicate a deleted final or initial consonant.

Column 10: S/I   The child's production is labeled as spontaneous (S) or imitated (I). If more detailed information is desired, the examiner can specify cued (C) or delayed imitation (DI).

Column 11: PCC: Child   The number of consonants correct for the child is entered here. Remember to include medial consonants that occur in two- and three-syllable words.

Column 13   Notes includes comments on the child's production, as needed. For example., assimilation, vowel error, or change in target word.

The next step is to enter summary numbers in the bottom row, based on the data in Columns 1, 4, 5, 11, 12:

- **Column 1** shows the number of words produced by the child.
- **Column 5** shows # of Word Structure Matches/# words produced.
- **Column 11** shows the Percentage of Consonants Correct (PCC) for the child's productions.
- **Column 12** shows the PCC for the target words.

IMPORTANT: If the child does not respond to an item, entries are labeled **NR**. If an item was not tested, entries are labeled **NT**.

Figure 3.2 shows an example of the entries for 20 words, with both the target and the child's productions.

Summarizing Data at the Bottom of the Word List   A brief summary of the entries in the table above (in Figure 3.2) yields the following measures for this set of words. This information will later be entered on the summary page of your test form.

a. **Total number** of target words in the sample: **19** (the list had 20 words but one word was not tested: **NT**).

b. **Total number** of words produced by the child: **17**.

c. **Number of words** for which the *word structure* of the child's production (based on the IPA in Column 3) matched the *word structure* of the target (shown in Column 4): **10** (see bottom of Column 5). (For this sample the WSM is 10 words out of 17 words produced, or 58.8%; this number is entered on the Summary page.)

d. **Word-initial consonants** in the child's productions: Column 7.

e. **Word-final consonants** in the child's productions: Column 9.

f. Total number of consonants in the child's productions that were **correct** (the sum of entries in Column 11) when compared to the target form. The **total number of consonants correct** for this set of words is **28.**

g. Total number of consonants in the target words (Column 12). The **total number of target consonants** for this set of words is **40**. NOTE: Words not produced by the child (2 entries with NR) and words not tested by the examiner (1 entry with NT) are not included in the calculation of PCC Target. These are indicated on the analysis form by a slash in Column 12.

The totals in Columns 11 and 12 yield a **PCC for this set of words** of **70%** (28/40).

Examples of completed forms are presented in Appendices 3.3 and 3.4.

Data Entry for the PEEPS Screener Word List   The PEEPS Screener contains a list of 20 words selected from the PEEPS Word List. Clinicians may choose to administer the Screener to determine if more in-depth assessment is warranted or if there is limited time.

Analysis of the children's production for the Screener is identical to the analyses described above for the full PEEPS analysis, and the Summary Analysis page is the same. If the child exhibits any of the following differences from what would be expected given the child's age (refer to *PEEPS Profiles* in Chapter 6), the full PEEPS protocol should be administered:

- Limited phonetic inventory
- Unusual errors; i.e., initial consonant deletion, glottal replacement, backing, and deletion of stressed syllables
- Frequent vowel errors

COL. 1	2	3	4	5	6	7	8	9	10	11	12	13
Word	IPA: Target	IPA: Child	WS Target	WSM	Initial C: Target	Initial C: Child	Final C: Target	Final C: Child	S/I	PCC: Child	PCC: Target	Notes
cow	kaʊ	kaʊ	CV	1	k	k			s	1	1	
moo	mu	mu	CV	1	m	m			s	1	1	
dog	dag	da	CVC	0	d	d	g	--	s	1	2	
woof	wʊf	wʊf	CVC	1	w	w	f	f	s	2	2	
finger	fɪŋgɚ	NT	CVCCV	NT	f	NT			NT	NT	3̶	
banana	bənænə	nænæna	CVCCV	0	b	n			s	2	3	Syl del.
fish(y)	fɪʃ(i)	fɪʃi	CVC(V)	1	f	f	(ʃ)		s	2	2	CVCV target
kitty(cat)	kɪt/di(kæt)	kikæʔ	CVCV(CVC)	0	k	k	(t)	ʔ	s	2̶(4)	Note [ʔ]
puppy	pʌpi	pʌpi	CVCV	1	p	p			s	2	2	
sheep	ʃip	ʃip	CVC	1	ʃ	t	p	p	s	1	2	
chicken	tʃɪkən	tsɪkən	CVCVC	1	tʃ	ts	n	n	s	2	3	Note [ts-]
bug	bʌg	NR	CVC	NR	b	NR	g	NR	NR	NR	2̶	
elephant	ɛləfət	ɛlfət	VCVCVCC	0			nt	t	1	3	4	
monkey	mʌŋki	mʌŋki	CVCCV	0	m	m			s	2	3	
lion	laɪ(j)ən	jaɪən	CV(C)VC	1	l	j	n	n	s	1	2	
foot	fʊt	fʊt	CVC	1	f	f	t	t	s	2	2	
cheese	tʃiz	NR	CVC	NR	tʃ	NR	z	NR	NR	NR	2̶	
hair	hɛɹ	hɛ	CVC	0	h	h	ɹ	--	s	1	2	
hand	hænd	hɛn	CVCC	0	h	h	nd	n	s	2	3	Note V
mouth	maʊθ	maʊf	CVC	1	m	m	θ	f	1	1	2	Note V
# words produced by child/ # words possible		17/19	# match	10/17					Total PCC	28	40	

Figure 3.2. An example of the entries (both target and child) for 20 words.

Completing the Summary Analysis Page

After completing data entry and analysis on the Word List page(s), you will complete the Summary Analysis Page. In the form, this page includes participant information and summaries of the independent and relational analyses derived from the word list on the next two pages of the forms. Similarly, the summary page for the PEEPS Screener is based on the independent and relational analyses derived from the 20 screener words.

Participant Information   The following information regarding participants and the testing session is entered:

a. Child's name. date of birth, date tested, test age, gender, and examiner

b. Number of words produced/number of words tested. Remember that word targets that were Not Tested are NOT included in the total number of possible words.

c. A section for *Notes* about the test session

Independent Analysis: Consonant Inventory and Word/Syllable Shapes   In this section, the consonants and consonant clusters produced in word-initial and word-final position are noted (circled on the list of consonants). Consonants that occur in the child's productions but *do not appear* on the list are also included. In Figure 3.2, the child produced the word *lion* as [jaɪən] with initial [j-] and *chicken* with the alveolar affricate [ts-]; in addition, the glottal stop [ʔ] occurs as the final consonant in the child's production of *kittycat:* [kikæʔ]. These consonants do not appear on the lists of PEEPS consonants, as none of the PEEPS words begins with [j-] or with [ts-] (an alveolar affricate, not a cluster) and none ends with a glottal stop. Thus, [j-] and [ts-] should be added to the list of initial consonants and [ʔ] should be added to the list of word-final consonants. The total number of *different consonants* in word-initial and word-final positions is entered, including those listed as "other."

Independent Analysis: Sound Classes   In this section, consonants occurring in word-initial and word-final positions are summarized in terms of **place and manner classes.**

• For **manner of articulation:**

  • 6 classes are listed for word-initial consonants and 5 classes for word-final consonants; classes occurring in the child's productions are circled and the total number of classes is entered.

• For **place of articulation:**

  • 7 classes are listed for word-initial consonants and 6 classes for word-final consonants; classes occurring in the child's productions are circled and the total number of classes is entered.

Independent Analysis: Word and Syllable Shapes   This section has two elements:

1. Number of syllables in the child's words

2. Word shape: presence/absence of final consonants; initial consonant clusters; final consonant clusters

Relational Analysis, Accuracy: Word Structure Match   To determine the percentage of WSM, the information from the bottom of Column 5 on pages 3–5 (or page 7 for the Screener Word List) is summed. The total is shown as the **#WSM/# Words Produced** and then converted to a percentage.

Relational Analysis, Accuracy: Percent Consonants Correct   PCC is based on a sum of the numbers appearing at the bottom of Columns 11 (PCC: Child) and 12 (PCC: Target on pages 3–5)

(or page 7 for the Screener Word List). The total is shown as **PCC: Child/PCC: Target** and then converted to a percentage.

Relational Analysis: Number of Syllables   The summary page uses a **Yes/No** format to indicate if the child's production matches the target in terms of **number of syllables.**

Relational Analysis: Red Flags   This section lists patterns that may be considered "red flags" (i.e., patterns that are unusual in the productions of children with typical phonological development).

From the Independent Analysis, the clinician would note if the word-final phonetic inventory was larger than the word-initial phonetic inventory. Red flags noted from the Relational Analysis would include the presence of unusual vowel errors, atypical consonant substitutions or deletions. While a child may produce some of these errors, a red flag would be indicated if these unusual or atypical errors occurred with a high frequency of around 50% occurrence.

CLINICAL CONSIDERATIONS

In this section, clinical considerations relative to testing and intervention are addressed. With regard to testing, children with very limited vocabularies are considered, as well as administering PEEPS remotely via telepractice or telehealth. Additional testing considerations are included in Chapter 4, which discusses assessment of toddlers who are multilingual. A section on developmentally appropriate intervention approaches is also included in Chapter 4.

Testing Considerations

In order for the examiner to complete the independent and relational analyses in PEEPS, the child needs to produce a minimum number of the PEEPS words. Specifically, a sample of at least 10 words must be elicited. In the PEEPS data collected on typically developing children, there were a few children at 18 and 21 months who did not meet that criterion. It is recommended that if a child produces fewer than 10 words on PEEPS, the clinician should bring the child back for testing in 4–6 weeks. The clinician can also request that parents or caregivers fill out the expressive word list from MacArthur-Bates Communicative Development Inventories, Second Edition (Fenson et al., 2007).

Remote Administration of PEEPS

Administration of PEEPS through telepractice requires adaptation to elicit the stimulus words and obtain a high-quality audio recording of the child for transcription. We have adapted elicitation in two ways. First, to preserve child manipulation of the toys, we sent families a set of toys to use during the assessment session. The parent who accompanied the child during the session was trained on how to present the toys by the clinician who guided the elicitation through an online session using a program like Zoom. Second, when sending the toys was not possible, we used a document camera attached to the computer so that the clinician could present the toys and manipulate them during the Zoom session. (A document camera is an updated digital version of an opaque projector that allows one to display objects in detail. Several basic models of document cameras are available on Amazon for less than $100.) The clinician could hide or manipulate the toys to keep the child's interest. Parents were encouraged to show excitement and assist in maintaining the child close to the screen. The optimal position for the child was on the parent's lap or in a highchair.

Obtaining a high-quality recording was another challenge in the telepractice environment. The options go from high- to low-tech and were determined in consultation with the parent before the session. We used LENA recorders positioned in vests worn by the child for the best recordings, but this option was not available for general clinical use. Some children were willing to wear a headset with microphone and that provided good audio fidelity. As an alternative, we did have parents record the session on their iPhone; however, any external recorder could be used. The best recordings were obtained when the parent held the phone near the child's face. This audio recording could be used along with the Zoom recording during the transcription process.

SUMMARY

In this chapter, information was provided on administering and completing the PEEPS test, including how to assemble the toys/objects for the test, obtaining a sample, and completing independent and relational analyses on the child's production of the test words. In Chapter 4, clinicians will be guided in how to interpret the findings from the independent and relational analyses. Important in the administration and interpretation of the results are cultural and linguistic considerations, including assessing multilingual toddlers. Finally, appropriate intervention approaches will be reviewed if intervention is recommended based on PEEPS results.

PEEPS Word List: Semantic Categories

The chart below shows the PEEPS words organized in semantic categories. Use this chart to plan how you will elicit each word. Note that in some cases, there is more than one way to elicit the word. Choose what is most practical based on the materials you have available in your setting. For example

- To elicit the word *hair*, you could point to hair on the baby doll (if applicable) or point to your own hair or the child's hair.

- To elicit the word *spoon*, you could point to the picture of a spoon in *A Book of Things*, or use an actual spoon if you have one on hand.

Words in the left column that are marked with an asterisk (*) are acquired between ages 22 and 24 months. For a few words, alternatives that are appropriate for children who speak British/Australian/New Zealand English are shown in italics.

	Use toy/object to elicit word.	Point to body part (on self, child, or baby doll) to elicit word.	Use gesture/action to elicit word.	Use *A Book of Things* to elicit word.
Baby/Body Parts For this category, "use toy or object" refers to the baby doll with accessories. The doll may be used to elicit *belly button*, *tongue*, and/or *hair* if these are included on the doll. The doll and blanket may be used to elicit *peek-a-boo*.				
baby	✓			
ear	✓	✓		
finger	✓	✓		
foot*	✓	✓		
tummy*	✓	✓		
hand	✓	✓		
mouth	✓	✓		
nose	✓	✓		
toe	✓	✓		
belly button		✓		
tongue*		✓		
hair		✓		
peek-a-boo	✓		✓	
bib*	✓			
hat	✓			
doll*	✓			
shoe	✓	✓		
sock*	✓	✓		
diaper *(nappy)*	✓			
blanket	✓			

Baby/Body Parts For this category, "use toy or object" refers to the baby doll with accessories. The doll may be used to elicit *belly button*, *tongue*, and/or *hair* if these are included on the doll. The doll and blanket may be used to elicit *peek-a-boo*.			
	Use toy/object to elicit word.	Point to body part (on self, child, or baby doll) to elicit word.	Use gesture/action to elicit word.	Use *A Book of Things* to elicit word.
comb*	✓			
bottle	✓			

Animals			
	Use toy/object to elicit word.	Point to body part (on self, child, or baby doll) to elicit word.	Use gesture/action to elicit word.	Use *A Book of Things* to elicit word.
fish	✓			
bird	✓			
cow	✓			
moo	✓			
mouse*	✓			
kitty	✓			
duck	✓			
quack	✓			
dog	✓			
puppy	✓			
woof	✓			
pig	✓			
chicken	✓			
lion*	✓			
elephant*	✓			
bug/beetle	✓			
monkey*	✓			
sheep*	✓			

Food A toy cup can be used to elicit the words *juice*, *cup*, and *drink*.			
	Use toy/object to elicit word.	Point to body part (on self, child, or baby doll) to elicit word.	Use gesture/action to elicit word.	Use *A Book of Things* to elicit word.
juice	✓			
cup	✓			
drink	✓		✓	
banana				✓

	Use toy/object to elicit word.	Point to body part (on self, child, or baby doll) to elicit word.	Use gesture/action to elicit word.	Use *A Book of Things* to elicit word.
Food A toy cup can be used to elicit the words *juice*, *cup*, and *drink*.				
cheese				✓
cookie (biscuit)				✓
spoon				✓
Miscellaneous A toy truck can be used to elicit the words *truck*, *go*, and *stop*. A flashlight can be used to elicit the words *light* and *off*.				
truck	✓			
go	✓			
stop*	✓			
light	✓		✓	
off	✓		✓	
ball				✓
balloon				✓
soap*				✓
rock*				✓
zipper*				✓
train*				✓
watch*				✓
block*				✓

Examples of Toys Used to Elicit PEEPS Words

Below are sample photos of the toys that can be collected to represent the PEEPS words. See Chapter 3 for additional guidance on toy selection.

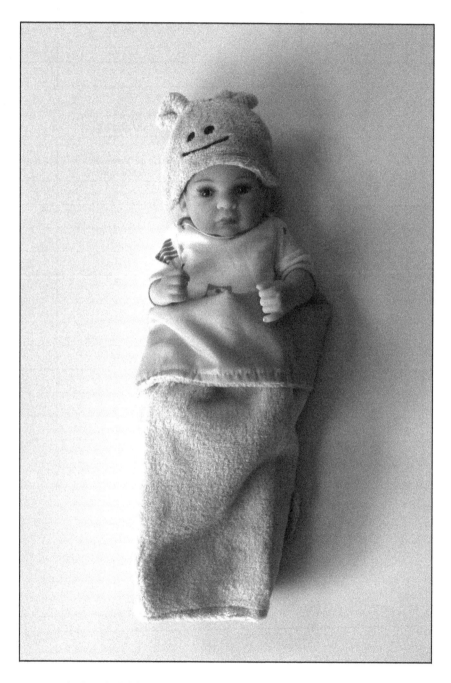

baby, doll, blanket, hat, hands, ear, finger, mouth, nose

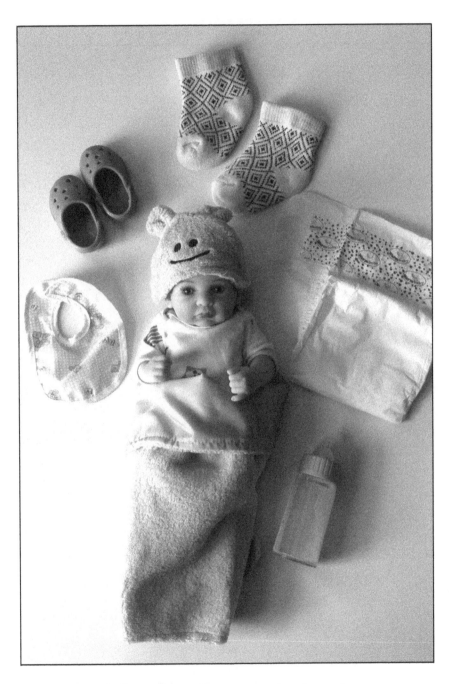

baby, doll, ear, finger, foot, tummy, hand, mouth, nose, blanket, hat, bib, shoes, socks, diaper (*nappy*), bottle

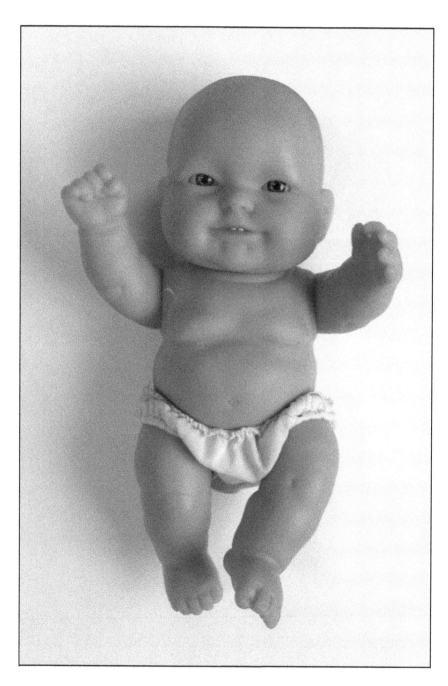

baby, doll, diaper (*nappy*), ear, finger, foot, tummy, hand, mouth, nose, belly button

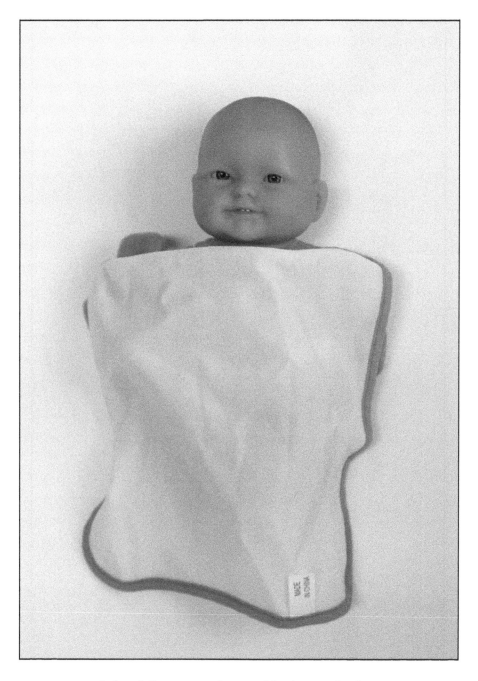

baby, doll, ear, mouth, nose, blanket, peek-a-boo

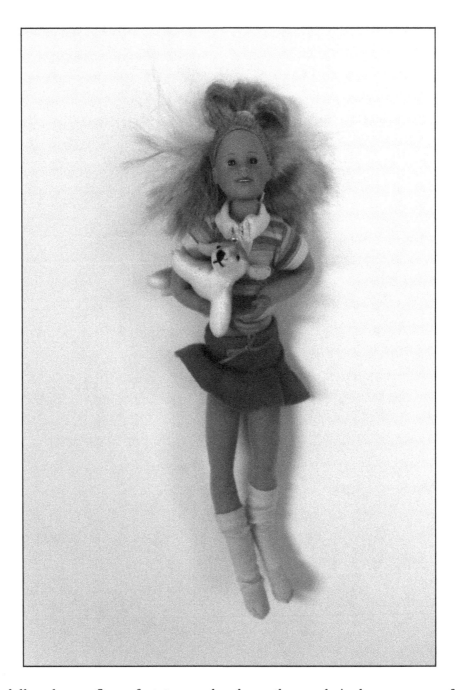

doll, socks, ear, finger, foot, tummy, hand, mouth, nose, hair, dog, puppy, woof

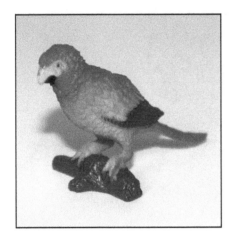

bird

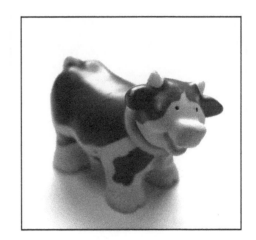

cow, moo

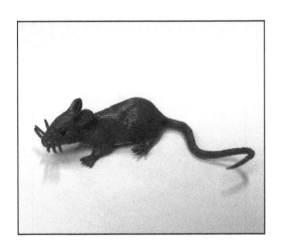

mouse

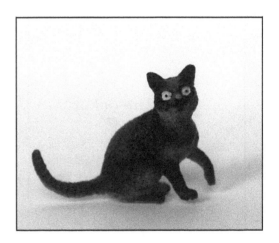

kitty

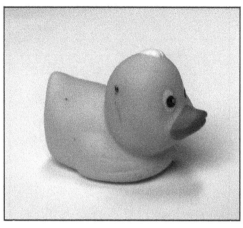

duck, quack

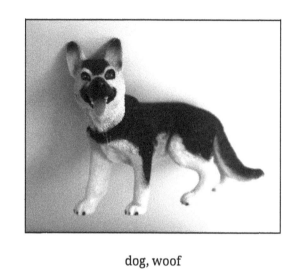

dog, woof

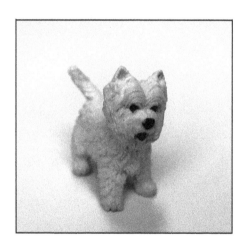

puppy, woof

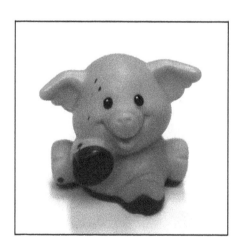

pig

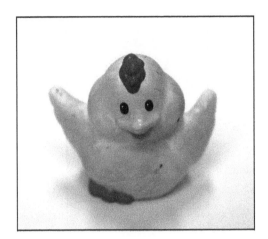

chicken

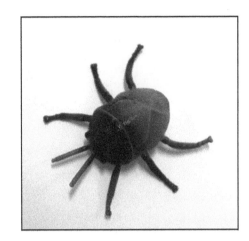

bug, beetle

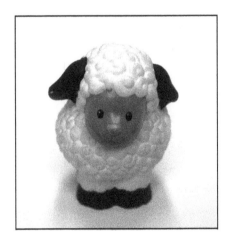

sheep

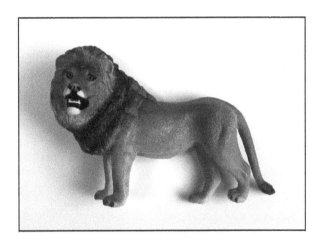

lion

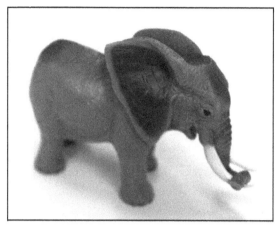

elephant

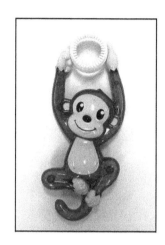

monkey

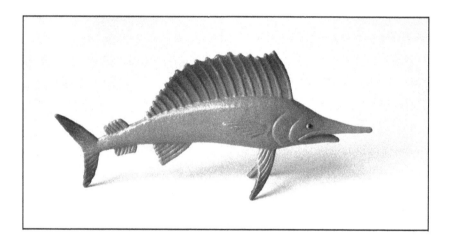

fish

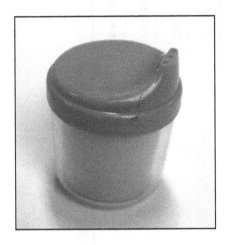

juice, cup, drink

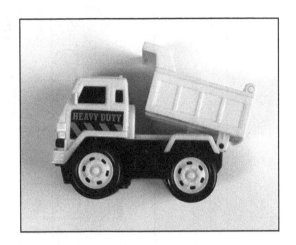

truck, go, stop

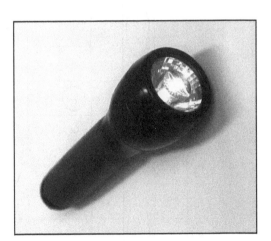

light, off

Sample Completed PEEPS Analysis Form: Hudson

The following pages show a sample completed PEEPS form for Hudson, a 21-month-old boy.

PEEPS Summary Analysis and Word List

peeps

Child's name: Hudson	Test age (months): 21	# Words Produced:	NOTES
Date of birth (Y/M/D): 2021/1/3	Gender: male		8 words: Not Tested (NT); 22 words: No Response (NR)
Date tested (Y/M/D): 2023/1/12	Examiner: ALW	30 / 52	Frequent final consonant deletion

Independent Analysis

Circle consonants and consonant clusters produced in each word position. Add consonants and clusters produced but not listed.

Consonant Inventory

Word-Initial Consonants	(p)	(b)	(t)	(d)	(k)	g	(f)	(s)	z	ʃ	tʃ	dʒ	(m)	(n)	l	ɹ	(w)	(h)	Other: n/a	Total: 11
Word-Initial Clusters	bl-	tɹ-	dɹ-	kw-	sp-	st-												Other: n/a	Total: 0
Word-Initial Manner	(Stop)	(Fricative)	Affricate	(Nasal)	Liquid	(Glide)								# Manner Classes: 4
Word-Initial Place	(Labial/labiodental)	(Alveolar/interdental)	Palatal	(Velar)	(Glottal)									# Places: 5
Word-Final Consonants	p	b	t	d	k	g	f	(s)	z	ʃ	tʃ	m	(n)	ŋ	l	ɹ		Other: n/a	Total: 2
Word-Final Clusters	-nd	-nt	-ŋk														Other: n/a	Total: 0
Word-Final Manner	Stop	(Fricative)	Affricate	(Nasal)	Liquid									# Manner Classes: 2
Word-Final Place	Labial/labiodental	(Alveolar/interdental)	Palatal	Velar										# Places: 1

Word and Syllable Shapes: Circle those that occur. **Number of syllables:** (1) (2) 3

Presence of: (Final consonant(s))   Initial consonant cluster   Final consonant cluster

Relational Analysis

Accuracy		Number of Syllables	
# WS Match / # Words Produced:	6 / 30	2-syllable	(Y) / N
PCC Child / PCC Target:	28 / 62	3-syllable	Y / (N)
WSM: 20 %			
PCC: 45.1 %			

Red Flags (See Manual for examples.)

WF inventory substantially > WI inventory	Y / (N)
Unusual Vowel Errors	Y / (N)
Atypical Consonant Substitutions	Y / (N)
Atypical Deletions	Y / (N)

(continued)

APPENDIX 3.3 (continued)

 peeps

Word	IPA: Target	IPA: Child	WS Target	WSM	Initial C: Target	Initial C: Child	Final C: Target	Final C: Child	S/I	PCC: Child	PCC: Target	Notes
cow	kaʊ	NT	CV	NT	k	NT			NT	NT	~~1~~	
moo	mu	NT	CV	NT	m	NT			NT	NT	~~1~~	
dog	dag	da	CVC	0	d	d	g	--	1	1	2	
woof	wʊf	fʊfʊ	CVC	0	w	f	f	--	S	1	2	*Target: woof-woof*
duck(y)	dʌk(i)	dʌ	CVC(V)	0	d	d	(k)	--	S	1	2	
quack	kwæk	NR	CCVC	NR	kw	NR	k	NR	NR	NR	~~3~~	
fish(y)	fɪʃ(i)	NT	CVC(V)	NT	f	NT	(ʃ)	NT	NT	NT	~~2~~	
bird	bɚd	bʊ	CVC	0	b	b	d	--	S	1	2	
kitty (cat)	kɪt/di (kæt)	kæ	CVCV(CVC)	0	k	k	(t)	--	S	1	2 ~~(4)~~	
puppy	pʌpi	pʌpi	CVCV	1	p	p			1	2	2	
*mouse	maʊs	ma	CVC	0	m	m	s	--	S	1	2	
pig(gy)	pɪg(i)	pɪ	CVC(V)	0	p	p	(g)	--	S	1	2	
*sheep	ʃip	NR	CVC	NR	ʃ	NR	p	NR	NR	NR	~~2~~	
chicken	tʃɪkən	NR	CVCVC	NR	tʃ	NR	n	NR	NR	NR	~~3~~	
bug	bʌg	NR	CVC	NR	b	NR	g	NR	NR	NR	~~2~~	
*elephant	ɛləfənt	NT	VCVCVCC	0			nt	NT	NT	NT	~~4~~	
*monkey	mʌŋki	NR	CVCCV	NR	m	NR	n	NR	NR	NR	~~3~~	
*lion	laɪ(j)ən	daɪ	CV(C)VC	0	l	d	n	--	S	0	2~~(3)~~	
baby	beɪbi	beɪbi	CVCV	1	b	b			S	2	2	
ear	ɪɹ	ɪ	VC	0			ɹ	--	S	0	1	
# words produced by child/# words possible	11/16	# match		2/11					Total PCC	11	21	

*indicates words acquired between 22–24 months

(continued)

APPENDIX 3.3 (continued)

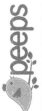
peeps

Word	IPA: Target	IPA: Child	WS Target	WSM	Initial C: Target	Initial C: Child	Final C: Target	Final C: Child	S/I	PCC: Child	PCC: Target	Notes
finger	fɪŋgɚ	NR	CVCCV	NR	f	NR			NR	NR	3	
*foot	fʊt	NR	CVC	NR	f	NR	t	NR	NR	NR	2	
hair	hɛɹ	hɛ	CVC	0	h	h	ɹ	⁓	S	1	2	
hand	hænd	NT	CVCC	NT	h	NT	nd	NT	NT	NT	3	
mouth	maʊθ	maʊ	CVC	0	m	m	θ	⁓	S	1	2	
nose	noʊz	noʊs	CVC	1	n	n	z	s	S	1	2	
toe(s)	toʊ(z)	NR	CV(C)	NR	t	NR	(z)	NR	NR	NR	1(2)	
*tummy	tʌmi	dʌ,j	CVCV	0	t	d			1	0	2	
*tongue	tʌŋ	NR	CVC	NR	t	NR	ŋ	NR	NR	NR	2	
belly button	bɛlibʌtən	NT	CVCVCVC	NT	b	NT	n	NT	NT	NT	5	
*soap	soʊp	NR	CVC	NR	s	NR	p	NR	NR	NR	2	
*comb	koʊm	koʊ	CVC	0	k	k	m	⁓	1	1	2	
blanket	blæŋkət	NR	CCVCCVC	NR	bl	NR	t	NR	NR	NR	5	
peek-a-boo	pikabu	NR	CVCVCV	NR	p	NR	l	⁓	NR	NR	3	
*doll	dɑl	dɑ	CVC	0	d	d	l	⁓	S	1	2	
shoe	ʃu	du	CV	1	ʃ	d			S	0	1	
*sock	sɑk	sɑ	CVC	0	s	s	k	⁓	1	1	2	
*zipper	zɪpɚ	NT	CVCV	NT	z	NT			NT	NT	2	
hat	hæt	hæ	CVC	0	h	h	t	⁓	1	1	2	
off	ɑf	NR	VC	NR		NR	f	NR	NR	NR	1	
# words produced by child/# words possible	9/17		# match	2/9					Total PCC	7	17	

*indicates words acquired between 22–24 months

(continued)

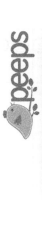

Word	IPA: Target	IPA: Child	WS Target	WSM	Initial C: Target	Initial C: Child	Final C: Target	Final C: Child	S/I	PCC: Child	PCC: Target	Notes
diaper	daɪpɚ	baɪbi	CVCV	1	d	b			1	0	2	
*bib	bɪb	NR	CVC	NR	b	NR	b	NR	NR	NR	~~2~~	
juice	dʒus	du	CVC	0	dʒ	d	s	--	S	0	2	
banana	bənænə	bænənə	CVCVCV	0	b	b			S	2	3	
cookie	kʊki	NR	CVCV	NR	k	NR			NR	NR	~~2~~	
cheese	tʃiz	tis	CVC	1	tʃ	t	z	s	S	0	2	
cup	kʌp	NR	CVC	NR	k	NR	p	NR	S	NR	~~2~~	
drink	drɪŋk	NR	CCVCC	NR	dr	NR	ŋk	NR	NR	NR	~~4~~	
bottle	bɑt/dɑl	bɑdə	CVCVC	0	b	b	l	vowel	NR	2	3	
spoon	spun	sun	CCVC	0	sp	s	n	n	1	2	3	
*train	treɪn	NR	CCVC	NR	tr	NR	n	NR	NR	NR	~~3~~	
truck	trʌk	NR	CCVC	NR	tr	NR	k	NR	NR	NR	~~3~~	
*stop	stɑp	NT	CCVC	NT	st	NT	p	NT	NT	NT	~~3~~	
go	goʊ	NR	CV	NR	g	NR			NR	NR	~~1~~	
light	laɪt	NR	CVC	NR	l	NR	t	NR	NR	NR	~~2~~	
balloon	bəlun	bu	CVCVC	0	b	b	n	--	1	1	3	
ball	bɑl	bɑ	CVC	0	b	b	l	--	S	1	2	
*rock	rɑk	wɑ	CVC	0	r	w	k	--	1	1	2	
*block	blɑk	NR	CCVC	NR	bl	NR	k	NR	NR	NR	~~3~~	
*watch	wɑtʃ	wɑ	CVC	0	w	w	tʃ	--	1	1	2	
# words produced by child/# words possible	10/19		# match	2/10					Total PCC	10	24	

*indicates words acquired between 22–24 months

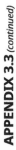

Sample Completed PEEPS Analysis Form: Yasmin

The following pages show a sample completed PEEPS form for Yasmin, a 30-month-old girl.

PEEPS Summary Analysis and Word List

Child's name: *Yasmin*	Test age *(months)*: 30	# Words Produced:
Date of birth *(Y/M/D)*: *2020/9/8*	Gender: *female*	
Date tested *(Y/M/D)*: *2023/3/9*	Examiner: *ALW*	*53 / 60*

NOTES

Independent Analysis

Circle consonants and consonant clusters produced in each word position. Add consonants and clusters produced but not listed.

Consonant Inventory

Word-Initial Consonants	(p)	(b)	(d)	(t)	(k)	g	(f)	(s)	z	(ʃ)	(tʃ)	(dʒ)	(m)	(n)	l · ɹ (w) (h)	Other: *j-*	Total: *14*
Word-Initial Clusters	bl-	tɹ-	dʒ-	(kw-)	sp-	st-										Other: *tw-*	Total: *2*
Word-Initial Manner	(Stop)				(Fricative)		(Affricate)			(Nasal)			(Liquid)		(Glide)	# Manner Classes: *5*
Word-Initial Place	(Labial/labiodental)						(Alveolar/interdental)			(Palatal)			(Velar)		(Glottal)	# Places: *6*
Word-Final Consonants	(p)	(b)	(d)	(t)	(k)	(g)	(f)	(s)	z	(ʃ)	(tʃ)	(m)	(n)	ŋ	(l) ɹ	Other: *n/a*	Total: *13*
Word-Final Clusters	-nd	-ŋk	-nt	-ŋk												Other: *n/a*	Total: *2*
Word-Final Manner	(Stop)						(Fricative)			(Affricate)			(Nasal)		(Liquid)	# Manner Classes: *5*
Word-Final Place	(Labial/labiodental)						(Alveolar/interdental)			(Palatal)			(Velar)			# Places: *5*

Word and Syllable Shapes: Circle those that occur.
Number of syllables: (1) (2) (3)

Presence of: (Final consonant(s)) (Initial consonant cluster) (Final consonant cluster)

Relational Analysis

Accuracy		Number of Syllables	
# WS Match / # Words Produced: *43 / 53*	**WSM:** *81.1 %*	2-syllable	(Y)/ N
PCC Child / PCC Target: *106 / 124*	**PCC:** *85.5%*	3-syllable	(Y)/ N

Red Flags (See Manual for examples.)	
WF inventory substantially > WI inventory	Y / (N)
Unusual Vowel Errors	Y / (N)
Atypical Consonant Substitutions	Y / (N)
Atypical Deletions	Y / (N)

(continued)

peeps

Word	IPA: Target	IPA: Child	WS Target	WSM	Initial C: Target	Initial C: Child	Final C: Target	Final C: Child	S/I	PCC: Child	PCC: Target	Notes
cow	kaʊ	kaʊ	CV	1	k	k			S	1	1	
moo	mu	mu	CV	1	m	m			S	1	1	
dog	dag	dag	CVC	1	d	d	g	g	S	2	2	
woof	wʊf	NR	CVC	NR	w	NR	f	NR	NR	NR	~~2~~	
duck(y)	dʌk(i)	dʌk	CVC(V)	1	d	d	(k)	k	S	2	2	
quack	kwæk	kwæk	CCVC	1	kw	kw	k	k	S	3	3	
fish(y)	fɪʃ(i)	fɪʃ	CVC(V)	1	f	f	(ʃ)	ʃ	S	2	2	
bird	bɝd	bʌd	CVC	1	b	b	d	d	1	2	2	
kitty (cat)	kɪt/di (kæt)	kʌdikæt	CVCV(CVC)	1	k	k	(t)	t	S	4	~~2~~(4)	
puppy	pʌpi	pʌpi	CVCV	1	p	p			S	2	2	
*mouse	maʊs	maʊs	CVC	1	m	m	s	s	S	2	2	
pig(gy)	pɪg(i)	pɪg	CVC(V)	1	p	p	(g)	g	S	2	2	
*sheep	ʃip	sip	CVC	1	ʃ	s	p	p	1	1	2	
chicken	tʃɪkən	tʃɪkən	CVCVC	1	tʃ	tʃ	n	n	S	3	3	
bug	bʌg	bʌg	CVC	1	b	b	g	g	S	2	2	
*elephant	ɛləfənt	fʌnt	VCVCVCC	0			nt	nt	S	3	4	
*monkey	mʌŋki	mʌŋki	CVCCV	1	m	m			S	3	3	
*lion	laɪ(j)ən	jaɪjən	CVC(j)VC	1	l	j	n	n	S	3	3	
baby	beɪbi	beɪbi	CVCV	1	b	b			S	2	2	
ear	ɪɹ	ɪə	VC	0	ɹ		ɹ	vowel	S	0	1	
# words produced by child/# words possible	19/20		# match	17/19					Total PCC	40	43	

*indicates words acquired between 22–24 months

(continued)

51

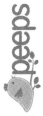 peeps

Word	IPA: Target	IPA: Child	WS Target	WSM	Initial C: Target	Initial C: Child	Final C: Target	Final C: Child	S/I	PCC: Child	PCC: Target	Notes
finger	fɪŋgɚ	fɪŋgə	CVCCV	1	f	f			1	3	3	
*foot	fʊt	fʊt	CVC	1	f	f	t	t	1	2	2	
hair	hɛɹ	hɛɜ	CVC	0	h	h	ɹ	vowel	S	1	2	
hand	hænd	hæn	CVCC	0	h	h	nd	n	S	2	3	
mouth	maʊθ	maʊf	CVC	1	m	m	θ	f	S	1	2	
nose	noʊz	noʊz	CVC	1	n	n	z	z	S	2	2	
toe(s)	toʊz	toʊz	CV(C)	1	t	t	(z)	z	S	2	~~1~~(2)	
*tummy	tʌmi	tʌmi	CVCV	1	t	t			S	2	2	
*tongue	tʌŋ	NR	CVC	NR	t	NR	ŋ	NR	NR	NR	~~2~~	
belly button	bɛlibʌtən	bɛdibʌtən	CVCVCVCVC	1	b	b	n	n	1	4	5	
*soap	soʊp	soʊp	CVC	1	s	s	p	p	S	2	2	
*comb	koʊm	koʊm	CVC	1	k	k	m	m	S	2	2	
blanket	blæŋkɛt	bæŋkɛt	CCVCCVC	0	bl	b	t	t	S	4	5	
peek-a-boo	pikəbu	NR	CVCVCV	NR	p	NR			NR	NR	~~3~~	
*doll	dɑl	dɑl	CVC	1	d	d	l	l	S	2	2	
shoe	ʃu	ʃu	CV	1	ʃ	ʃ			S	1	1	
*sock	sɑk	sɑk	CVC	1	s	s	k	k	1	2	2	
*zipper	zɪpɚ	dɪpə	CVCV	1	z	d			1	1	2	
hat	hæt	hæt	CVC	1	h	h	t	t	S	2	2	
off	ɑf	ɑf	VC	1			f	f	S	1	1	
# words produced by child/# words possible	18/20		#match	15/18					Total PCC	36	42	

*indicates words acquired between 22–24 months

(continued)

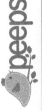

Word	IPA: Target	IPA: Child	WS Target	WSM	Initial C: Target	Initial C: Child	Final C: Target	Final C: Child	S/I	PCC: Child	PCC: Target	Notes
diaper	daɪpɚ	daɪpə	CVCV	1	d	d			S	2	2	
*bib	bɪb	bɪb	CVC	1	b	b	b	b	S	2	2	
juice	dʒus	dʒus	CVC	1	dʒ	dʒ	s	s	S	2	2	
banana	bənænə	ənænæ	CVCVCV	0	b	Del.			S	2	3	*Syl Del*
cookie	kʊki	kɔki	CVCV	1	k	k			S	2	2	
cheese	tʃiz	tʃɪs	CVC	1	tʃ	tʃ	z	s	S	1	2	
cup	kʌp	kʌp	CVC	1	k	k	p	p	S	2	2	
drink	drɪŋk	dɪŋk	CCVCC	0	dr	d	ŋk	ŋk	S	3	4	
bottle	bɑtl/bɑdl	bɑdu	CVCVC	0	b	b	l	vowel	1	2	3	
spoon	spun	NR	CCVC	NR	sp	NR	n	NR	NR	NR	~~3~~	
*train	treɪn	NR	CCVC	NR	tr	NR	n	NR	NR	NR	~~3~~	
truck	trʌk	twʌk	CCVC	1	tr	tw	k	k	S	2	3	*Init CC: [tw]*
*stop	stɑp	NR	CCVC	NR	st	NR	p	NR	NR	NR	~~3~~	
go	goʊ	NR	CV	NR	g	NR			NR	NR	~~1~~	
light	laɪt	jaɪt	CVC	1	l	j	t	t	S	1	2	
balloon	bəlun	bun	CVCVC	0	b	b	n	n	S	2	3	
ball	bɑl	bɑl	CVC	1	b	b	l	l	S	2	2	
*rock	rɑk	wɑk	CVC	1	r	w	k	k	S	1	2	
*block	blɑk	bɑk	CCVC	0	bl	b	k	k	1	2	3	
*watch	wɑtʃ	wɑtʃ	CVC	1	w	w	tʃ	tʃ	1	2	2	
# words produced by child/# words possible	16/20		# match	11/16					Total PCC	30	39	

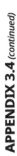

*indicates words acquired between 22–24 months

4 Analyzing and Interpreting Data

The previous chapter described how to complete the independent and relational analyses in PEEPS. In this chapter, information is provided on how to interpret the analysis results. Cultural and linguistic considerations will also be discussed. Finally, the chapter will present recommendations for determining next steps in terms of designing developmentally appropriate intervention.

INTERPRETING THE ANALYSIS RESULTS

Using the information from the independent and relational analyses, clinicians can make decisions about whether the child's phonological development is typical or atypical. Stoel-Gammon and Stone (1991) and Williams and Stoel-Gammon (2016) reported on the "critical elements" that you would expect to see in typically developing children at 18, 24, and 36 months. Based on an independent analysis, the critical elements encompass inventory, in terms of place and manner, and word structure at each of these three age periods, as summarized in Table 4.1.

Red Flags

In addition to these critical elements based on an independent analysis, Stoel-Gammon and Stone (1991) and Williams and Stoel-Gammon (2016) noted "red flags" from a relational analysis that could indicate atypical development. These may indicate unusual/atypical phonological patterns in the child's productions. Possible red flags are listed in Table 4.2 and include both atypical consonant substitutions and deletions.

In identifying atypical phonological development, Williams and Elbert (2003) described the presence of a cluster of behaviors using independent and relational analyses. Both quantitative and qualitative differences generally occur. For example, quantitative differences often include a smaller phonetic inventory and lower Percentage of Consonants Correct (PCC) score, along with a smaller lexicon. Qualitatively, atypical error patterns, greater sound variability, and simpler word structures are noted.

It is important to note that a single occurrence or relatively few occurrences of one of the red flags noted above is not sufficient evidence on its own to indicate atypical development. In toddlers, normal variations in productions are expected. Therefore, to be of concern, presence of one or more of these red flags should occur with relative frequency.

Dos and Don'ts

PEEPS provides a comprehensive and developmentally appropriate assessment of early phonological skills in young children 18–36 months of age. The independent analysis provides

Table 4.1. Critical elements at age 18, 24, and 36 months

	Typical Development		
Age	18 months	24 months	36 months
	Presence of: • Supraglottal consonants (e.g., consonants produced above or anterior to the glottis)–*PLACE* • A labial-lingual distinction (e.g., [b] and [d])–*PLACE* • An oral-nasal distinction (e.g., [m] and [b])–*MANNER* • Simple CV syllables (e.g., [dɑ] for "dog")	Presence of: • A range of manner classes, including stops, nasals, glides, and fricatives–*MANNER* • Labial and lingual consonants (e.g., [b] and [d])–*PLACE* • Open and closed syllables that can be combined to make disyllabic words	Adult sound system is fully represented in terms of sound classes (*PLACE* and *MANNER*) and word shapes (*WORD STRUCTURE*)
	Atypical Development		
	Lacking one or more of these critical elements	Smaller inventory of consonants and syllable structures, specifically: • Inventory limited to front stops and nasals and 1 or 2 glides • Syllable shapes restricted to open syllables (e.g., CV or CVCV)	Gaps in the system, such as failure to develop a fricative sound class or to develop syllable shapes beyond the simple CV

information about the size and nature of the child's phonetic inventory in terms of place, manner, and voicing. Clinicians will also have information regarding the syllable or word structure of the child's productions. As noted in Chapter 3, this information is helpful in examining the child's phonological capabilities in relation to what would be expected for a young child. Finally, the PEEPS relational analysis provides detailed information regarding the accuracy of the child's productions as well as the type of error patterns produced (i.e., typical or atypical). Together, the independent and relational analyses provide a composite of the child's phonological skills that can identify if there are any red flags noted in their phonological development. Profiles of typical development at 18, 24, 30, and 36 months provide further comparison for clinicians to make a diagnosis of the child's phonological development.

When making this diagnosis, it is important to keep certain dos and don'ts in mind. Clinicians *should not* use PEEPS results to assess communication abilities or skills PEEPS was not designed to measure. Additionally, clinicians *should* consider PEEPS results in context along with other sources of information about the child's communication development.

Don't Use PEEPS to Assess Abilities It Is Not Designed to Assess　　While PEEPS gives a comprehensive description of the child's phonological skills, it does not assess other aspects of communication development, such as social-pragmatic, syntactic, or semantic abilities. Only limited information on any voice or fluency issues may be noted from interactions with the child during PEEPS administration or collection of a language sample. Finally, clinicians cannot make any judgments regarding a child's hearing status from administering PEEPS. A puretone and tympanometry screening is recommended at all initial diagnostic assessments.

Table 4.2. Red Flags for atypical phonological development

Atypical Consonant Substitutions	Atypical Deletions
• Substitution of glottal consonants (e.g., [h] for /d/: [haʊ] for "down") • Backing (e.g., [k] for /t/: [kæʊ] for "tail")	• Initial consonant deletion (e.g., [aʊ] for "cow") • Deletion of stressed syllables (e.g., [di] for "candy")

Do Gather Additional Information to Supplement PEEPS Data   PEEPS' assessment of phonological development represents a single aspect of a full evaluation of a child's speech and language development. As noted previously, there is a close relationship between lexical and phonological development in toddlers. Therefore, gathering information on the child's vocabulary size, both in terms of production and comprehension, is another important piece of the puzzle in understanding the child's speech and language skills. We recommend administering the *MacArthur Communicative Development Inventories (CDIs): Words and Sentences*, within the CDI English Set, *Third Edition* (Marchman et al., 2023) to assess a child's vocabulary development. We also recommend collecting a sample of the child's spontaneous connected speech to examine overall intelligibility, but also to see how the child uses language to initiate and respond in communicative interactions. Case history (medical, developmental, familial) information is also important to determine if additional factors may be contributing to the child's development, including a history of ear infections as well as a family history of speech and/or language disorders.

Cultural and Linguistic Considerations

In this section, information is provided regarding considerations in administering PEEPS to children who are from linguistically and culturally diverse backgrounds, as well as to multilingual children. Considerations include the child's familiarity with the testing situation and with the activity of object labeling, whether the child uses a dialect of English other than General American English, and finally, the value of dynamic assessment.

Cross-Cultural Assessment   Carter and colleagues (2005) discussed a number of issues in the development of cross-cultural assessments of speech and language for children. Of those they noted, *familiarity with the testing situation* is relevant to administering PEEPS to toddlers. Fortunately, toys help all children feel more comfortable in the test environment. As noted previously, grouping the toys into semantic categories helps with collecting the toys, but it is also helpful in moving through the PEEPS test items. Beginning with the farm animals is often best to make children feel more comfortable. Younger children, especially, often learn to say the sounds that the animals make earlier than they learn the names of the animals.

Peña and colleagues (Peña et al., 1992; Peña & Quinn, 1997) reported that object labeling is an unfamiliar activity that is not taught in the home or community to Puerto Rican children in the United States. If testing children from a culture where naming objects is not a familiar activity, the clinician can use the toys to play and describe and then ask the child to name the item. The cueing hierarchy used in PEEPS lends itself well to working with children not accustomed to naming objects.

Another consideration is testing children who speak a *dialect* different from General American English. This is less of a concern with PEEPS because the independent analysis does not judge the accuracy of the production, but it is important to note the child's dialect on the relational analysis as a difference rather than as an error. For example, a phonological characteristic of African American English (AAE) is production of the written symbol *th* in word-initial position is variably yet systematically produced with /d/. Therefore, a child who speaks AAE who named *thumb* as [dʌm] would not be considered to be making an error of stopping and voicing.

PEEPS can be used in *other English-speaking countries* but it is important to note the differences in word labels that exist. For example, the American words *diaper, cookie, cracker, kitty,* and *bug* are elicited as the British, Australian, or New Zealand English equivalents of *nappy, biscuit, biscuit, cat,* and *bug/beetle* respectively.

Finally, Carter et al. (2005) note the value of *dynamic assessment* in the development of assessments in cross-cultural situations. As dynamic assessment typically involves a sequence of testing that includes pretesting, a testing element, and post-testing to focus on what the child learns rather than what they know, this methodology is incorporated within the cueing hierarchy of PEEPS. Specifically, the clinician attempts to elicit the child's response spontaneously (similar to pre-testing) and then goes through a series of prompts including cueing, delayed imitation, and direct imitation (teaching element). If the child does not name the object following the sequence of prompts, the toy is put back in the cube (or sack) and given another opportunity to name (post-testing). The aim is to elicit as representative a sample as possible from the child; PEEPS is not a vocabulary test.

Multilingual Toddlers   Differences in phonetic and phonemic inventories across languages will require clinicians to incorporate additional steps to assess multilingual toddlers' speech, particularly if the clinician does not speak the same language. McLeod and colleagues (2017; p. 694) outlined several steps, including:

- Becoming familiar with the phonetic and phonologic characteristics of the language

- Using a parent or caregiver (or other native speaker) as an informant

- Recording the child's speech using high-quality audio and video equipment

In addition to these steps, Cronin and colleagues (2020) described a holistic communication assessment to assess the speech of 2- to 3-year-old children with cleft palate that included a number of measures in addition to the speech and language assessment. A holistic assessment involves a family-centered approach that considers the child's participation in daily life activities along with their strengths and includes information from parents, caregivers, other family members, and educators. Several of these additional measures would be beneficial to include with multilingual children, particularly when the clinician does not speak their language. Among these measures were a case history questionnaire and interview, which would provide information about languages spoken at home in addition to medical, developmental, and education information. The assessment also included observation of the child in their home, in childcare, and in the community to understand them in their daily life contexts. Cronin and colleagues also described a time-use diary (Australian Institute of Family Studies, 2006) in which parents complete a 24-hour record of their child's activities and movements in 15-minute increments. This diary gives the clinician unique information on the child's daily life in terms of child and family activities, as well as their priorities, in what the child does, who they do activities with, and where the child goes in a typical weekday. This holistic information not only provides information about the child's communication but can also help parents, family members, caregivers, and educators learn how to facilitate the child's speech if atypical development has been identified.

With regard to gathering and analyzing a speech sample, the clinician can use the PEEPS toys to elicit the child's single-word responses. As noted above, the clinician should include a parent, family member, or informant to assist them. McGregor and colleagues (1997) and McLeod et al. (2017) describe using a *family member contrastive analysis* to analyze the child's speech when the clinician is not familiar with the child's language(s). This involves recording the child's production of each PEEPS toy word in addition to asking the parent or other adult to produce the same word. In essence, the clinician is eliciting words from both the child and the adult to obtain the single-word sample. To assist the clinician in analyzing the child's phonological skills, the clinician can ask the family member to identify if the word was produced correctly or not, which will provide information for calculation of PCC and Word Structure Matches (WSM) for the relational analysis. Additionally, the clinician would transcribe both the child and adult's production and compare them to identify phonetic differences. A combination of these two methods will help the clinician analyze and evaluate the child's phonological skills.

Finally, McLeod and colleagues (2021) utilized an emergence approach described by Davis and Bedore (2013) to describe ambient phonology influences and cross-linguistic transfer in the phonology of two brothers (aged 5;6 and 3;10) in a three-generation Vietnamese-English family. The emergence approach views phonological acquisition as an interaction of physical and social interaction capacities between children and adults who scaffold a young child's general skills to acquire the complex knowledge of the sound system of a language. This generational speech analysis of family members provides an additional method for clinicians to utilize in assessing the phonology of multilingual children.

Other Cultural Considerations   The following additional suggestions from Carter et al. (2005) are beneficial considerations in creating culturally valid assessment procedures when administering PEEPS to culturally and linguistically diverse children:

- Enlist the assistance of the parent or caregiver to assist in the assessment procedures if needed. Utilizing familiar individuals from the child's ethnic group and language background is assumed to make testing adaptations most effective.

- Use assessment materials familiar to children in the local area. This includes selecting toys used in PEEPS. Simple but often overlooked items such as skin color of the baby doll used in PEEPS or types of bugs or fish could make a difference to children's understanding and participation in the assessment.

- When working with children who are unfamiliar with the testing situation, it may be helpful to include some practice items to help them become comfortable in the test environment and more readily interested in participating in the tasks.

DETERMINING NEXT STEPS

If the child is determined to have atypical or delayed phonological development, they will need speech sound intervention. The following section describes two evidence-based speech sound intervention approaches that have been specifically designed for young children: the Enhanced Milieu Teaching with Phonological Emphasis (EMT/PE) approach and the Stimulability approach.

Developmentally Appropriate Intervention

Early identification and intervention are critical because of long-term impacts on later aspects of development such as literacy and learning, as well the potential to negatively impact different aspects of children's lives, such as social interactions and peer relationships. Just as it is important to use a developmentally appropriate test to assess the early phonological skills of toddlers, it is equally important to implement a developmentally appropriate intervention approach for those children identified with atypical or delayed phonological skills. Williams and colleagues (2021) included chapters on interventions that are specifically designed for young children with emerging sound systems. Two approaches that are relevant for this clinical population include the Enhanced Milieu Teaching with Phonological Emphasis (EMT/PE) approach (Scherer et al., 2021) and the Stimulability approach (Miccio & Elbert, 1996; Miccio & Williams, 2021). A brief overview of each approach is provided below. Clinicians are encouraged to read the chapters on these approaches in *Interventions for Speech Sound Disorders in Children*, Second Edition (Williams et al., 2021) and view the video demonstrations provided with that text.

Enhanced Milieu Teaching With Phonological Emphasis   EMT/PE was developed for children under the age of 3 to address vocabulary and phonological skills in tandem. This approach aligns with the fact that lexical and phonological acquisition are closely associated. Components of the EMT/PE approach include selection of target words based on phonologic and vocabulary criteria. It utilizes prompting strategies (model, expand, requests, and recasts) in a responsive interaction and environmental arrangement aimed to promote engagement in play and communicative activities. The EMT-PE approach also includes extensive parent education to use environmental arrangement, responsiveness interactions, and milieu teaching procedures to prompt their child to imitate the target words.

Stimulability Approach   The Stimulability approach was developed for young children 2–4 years old who have very small phonetic inventories and are not stimulable for production of many or all of the sounds missing from their inventory. This approach is focused on increasing the child's stimulability skills, not acquisition of sounds. Therefore, it is a short-term, transitional intervention approach that typically lasts for only 12 sessions, but no longer than 12 weeks. Based on research on children's learning, the Stimulability approach encompasses seven important components, including the pairing of consonants with alliterative sound characters and hand/body motions for all consonants (both stimulable and non-stimulable). For example, "Zippy Zebra" is paired with the zipping coat hand motion. These sound character cards are incorporated within play-based turn-taking activities that are designed to maintain joint focus or joint attention and result in early communicative success that encourages vocal practice.

Similarities of these intervention approaches for toddlers with delayed or atypical phonological development include goals and activities that are developmentally appropriate. That is, both incorporate broad-based goals that are not phoneme-specific, as well as communication-focused activities that are play-based involving turn-taking. Finally, both approaches incorporate parents (particularly EMT/PE) and/or siblings (Stimulability).

Other Follow-Up

Depending on the findings from PEEPS, additional follow-up may be indicated with regard to further communication assessment of language, cognitive, and hearing abilities.

Once a child is identified as needing early intervention services, the family may request a report be shared with their child's pediatrician, as well as with their teacher if they are enrolled in an early childhood program. If the child is found eligible for early intervention (EI) services under the Individuals with Disabilities Education Improvement Act (IDEA) of 2004, Part C, which is the Program for Infants and Toddlers with Disabilities, an Individualized Family Service Plan (IFSP) is developed and generally includes an interdisciplinary team of the family, service coordinator, and intervention provider(s), which often includes the speech-language pathologist, and other therapies as indicated (e.g., occupational therapist and physical therapist). EI services under IDEA include infants and toddlers from birth to age 3 who have a congenital and/or developmental condition that has a probability of resulting in developmental delay. Under IDEA, EI begins at the point the child is referred to the Part C systems and typically ends when the child is 36 months old and transitions out of the system. According to McManus and colleagues (2020), receipt of actual services involves the joint responsibility of primary care, the EI team, and families.

SUMMARY

In this chapter, information was provided on how to interpret the PEEPS analysis that incorporates red flags that signal a delay in a child's phonological development. Important cultural and linguistic considerations were provided when testing children who speak a different dialect from General American English or who speak more than one language. Recommendations were also provided for creating culturally valid assessment procedures that incorporate dynamic assessment activities. Finally, two evidence-based intervention approaches were described that are specifically developed for late talkers (EMT/PE and Stimulability). In Chapter 5, PEEPS data will be presented for three children, ages 22–32 months, who present delayed, deviant, and typical phonological acquisition according to the Developmental Profiles that are provided for different age ranges.

5 | PEEPS in Practice: Interpreting Results Through Three Case Studies

This chapter will present case studies of three children who vary in age and phonological skills. These case studies illustrate the information that clinicians can obtain from PEEPS and how to compare the results to the PEEPS Profiles to determine if the child's phonological development is typical, delayed but following the expected developmental sequence, or delayed and atypical in developmental sequence.

Before presenting the case studies, it is useful to understand the phonological development of Late Talkers (LTs). As noted in Chapter 1, one of the target populations for PEEPS assessment is the group of children identified as LTs. Although the criteria for identifying LTs varies slightly from one study to another, these children all share one characteristic: acquisition of productive vocabulary is delayed. At 18 months, children with typical development have a productive vocabulary of about 50 words; by 24 months, the vocabulary increases substantially, with children producing 250–350 words. Children labeled as LTs fail to adhere to the expected vocabulary norms, with fewer than 10 words at 18 months and fewer than 50 words at 24 months.

Several studies of LTs indicate that their phonological development is also slow, with reduced phonetic inventories, limited word and syllable shapes, low intelligibility, and reduced accuracy (see Alt et al., 2021; Capone Singleton, 2018; Munro et al., 2021; Rescorla & Dale, 2013; Williams & Elbert, 2003). In some cases, the LTs "catch up" with their peers in terms of speech and language by age 3;0. In other cases, the delays continue and deviant patterns become apparent. The case studies presented in this chapter include PEEPS data from two children classified as LTs. Though both children exhibit slow phonological development, the profile of one child (Nick) follows the patterns documented for children with typical development; in contrast, the profile of the other child (Jane) displays a deviant course of development. Each of these cases is presented in the following sections.

CASE STUDY: NICK, AGE 22 MONTHS

Nick, a 22-month-old male, was an only child in a two-parent home where General American English (GAE) was the spoken language. His mother requested an assessment of his speech development due to concerns about his few spoken words and use of gestures and grunts to express his wants and needs.

An early version of PEEPS was administered in which Nick produced 22 words. The following is a summary of the independent and relational analyses on his productions of these words. A full transcript and analysis of Nick's productions are shown in Appendix 5.1 at the end of this chapter.

Independent Analysis

Findings from the independent analysis of Nick's speech productions were as follows.

Phonetic Inventory   Nick presented with a limited phonetic inventory that included primarily anterior stops [b, t, d], nasals [m, n], and glide [w] in the word-initial position. Place of production was primarily labial and alveolar. Nick produced one posterior consonant: fricative [ʃ]. With the exception of [t, ʃ], all word-initial consonants were voiced.

Word-finally, Nick produced 3 consonants in his inventory: [s, ɚ, ɹ], which included 3 different manners (fricative, liquid, stop) and 3 places of production (alveolar, palatal, and glottal). Two of the three word-final consonants were voiceless.

Syllable Structure   Nick's syllable structure was primarily simple and consisted of CVC and CV, with one CVCV ("baby"). He produced one word-final cluster (CVCC).

Summary of Independent Analysis

- 7 word-initial consonants; 3 word-final consonants
- Primarily voiceless labial and alveolar stops, nasals, glides with one voiceless alveolar fricative in word-final position
- Word-initial phonetic inventory is larger than word-final phonetic inventory
- Relatively complete vowel production across front, central, and back vowels
- Simple syllable structure

Relational Analysis

Findings from the relational analysis of Nick's speech productions were as follows.

Error Patterns   Word-initially, Nick primarily used the stops [b, d] which resulted in errors of voicing, fronting, and stopping. Another occasional error pattern was initial consonant deletion. Finally, cluster reduction was noted.

Word-finally, Nick frequently deleted final consonants. Also prevalent was the pattern of glottalization (production of a glottal stop for several consonants).

Accuracy: Percentage of Consonants Correct (PCC) = 37.5% accuracy

Word Shape (WS) Match: 59.1% match

Summary of Relational Analysis

- Developmental error patterns of voicing, fronting, stopping, final consonant deletion, and cluster reduction
- Initial consonant deletion and glottalization were also noted
- Reduced accuracy (37.5%) but matched word structure on 59.1% of words

Comparison to PEEPS Profile

Given Nick's age of 22 months, his phonological analysis was compared to the PEEPS Profile at 21 months. The comparison of his results to the 21-month Profile is summarized in Table 5.1.

Clinical Impression

Although Nick's PEEPS analysis reveals he has a smaller word-initial (7 consonants) and word-final inventory (3 consonants) compared to the 21-month profile (11 word-initial and 6.7 word-final consonants), it follows the expected acquisition of stops, nasals, and glides at labial and

Table 5.1. Comparison of Nick's phonological analysis to 21-month PEEPS Profile

	Nick's Analysis (age 22 months)	PEEPS Profile: 21 months
Vocabulary	Parent report of 30 words with no 2-word combinations	~ 125 words with 2-word combinations
PEEPS words produced	22 words	27.9 words
Phonetic Inventory		
Word-initial consonants	7	11
Word-final consonants	3	6.7
Manner classes	4 (primarily stops, nasals; 1 glide, 1 fricative)	3 (stop, nasal, glide)
Places of production	3 (primarily labial, alveolar; 1 palatal)	4 (labial, labiodental, alveolar, emerging: velar, glottal)
Word and syllable shapes	Simple: CVC, CV primarily (1 CVCV) 1 WF cluster	V, CV, CVCV (CVCVC); 0.6 different clusters WI; 0.3 WF
Accuracy/Match PCC WSM	37.5% 59.1%	58.3% 48.4%

alveolar places of production. His overall consonant accuracy was lower than the profile of a 21-month-old (PCC 37.5% compared to PCC 58.3%); however, his word shape match (WSM) was higher (WSM 59.1% compared to WSM 48.4%). With regard to Nick's error patterns, they generally reflected developmental errors expected at 2 years of age, though he exhibited occasional red flag errors (initial consonant deletion).

Based on these results, Nick presents a delay in his phonological development. Recommendations should be given to his parents for ways to stimulate and facilitate his phonological and lexical development with a follow-up re-evaluation in 3–6 months.

CASE STUDY: JANE, AGE 32 MONTHS

Jane, age 32 months, was the youngest of two children in a two-parent home where GAE was the only language spoken in the home. Her parents and pediatrician requested an evaluation due to concerns about Jane's slow speech and language development.

An early version of PEEPS was administered in which Jane produced 29 words. The following is a summary of the independent and relational analyses on her productions of these words. A full transcript and analysis of Jane's productions are shown in Appendix 5.2.

Independent Analysis

Findings from the independent analysis of Jane's speech productions were as follows.

Phonetic Inventory Jane presented with a limited phonetic inventory that included stop [d], nasals [m, n], and glides [w, j, h] in the word-initial position. Place of production was primarily labial and alveolar, with the palatal [j] and glottal [h] glides. All word-initial consonants were voiced with the exception of [h].

Word-finally, Jane did not produce any consonants.

Syllable Structure Jane's syllable structure was primarily simple and consisted of CV and CVCV. She did not produce any clusters word-initially or word-finally.

Summary of Independent Analysis

- 7 word-initial consonants; 0 word-final consonants

- Voiced alveolar stop, labial and alveolar nasals, labial and palatal and glottal glides

- Word-initial phonetic inventory is significantly larger than word-final phonetic inventory
- Relatively complete vowel production across front, central, and back vowels
- Simple syllable structure

Relational Analysis

Findings from the relational analysis of Jane's speech productions were as follows.

Error Patterns   Word-initially, Jane primarily used the stop [d], which resulted in errors of voicing, fronting, and stopping. Another common error pattern was gliding of liquids. Additionally, cluster reduction was noted. Word-finally, Jane consistently deleted final consonants.

Accuracy: PCC = 17.8% accuracy

WS Match: 27.6% match

Summary of Relational Analysis

- Developmental error patterns of voicing, fronting, stopping, gliding, final consonant deletion, and cluster reduction
- Significantly reduced accuracy (17.8%) and low word structure match (27.6%)

Comparison to PEEPS Profile

Given Jane's age of 32 months, her phonological analysis was compared to the PEEPS Profile at 33 months. The comparison of her results to the 33-month profile is summarized in Table 5.2.

Clinical Impression

As Jane's PEEPS analysis reveals, her phonetic inventory (7 consonants) is significantly smaller than expected compared to the PEEPS Profile for a 33-month-old (15 consonants), Jane also had with no word-final consonants (compared with the expected 12 word-final consonants in the 33-month-old profile). Although her inventory is significantly smaller, it follows the early acquisition of stops, nasals, and glides. Also notable was Jane's very low accuracy of consonant

Table 5.2.   Comparison of Jane's phonological analysis to 33-month PEEPS Profile

	Jane's Analysis (age 32 months)	PEEPS Profile: 33 months
Vocabulary	Parent report of 45 words with no 2-word combinations	> 1,000 words with multi-word utterances
PEEPS words produced	29 words	54.1 words
Phonetic Inventory		
Word-initial consonants	7	15
Word-final consonants	0	12.1
Manner classes	3 (stops, nasals, glides)	6 (stop, nasal, glide, fricative, affricate, liquid)
Places of production	4 (labial, alveolar, palatal, glottal)	6 (labial, labiodental, alveolar, palatal, velar, emerging: glottal)
Word and syllable shapes	Simple: CV, CVC, primarily; 1 CVCV No clusters WI or WF	V, CV, CVCV, CVCVC, CVCVCV, CCV; -VCC 3.9 different clusters WI; 3.2 WF (30 months)
Accuracy/Match PCC WSM	17.8% 27.6%	76.7% 75.6%

production (PCC of 17.8% compared to the expected PCC of 76.7%), as well as a significantly lower word shape match (WSM of 32.3% compared to the expected 75.6%). In addition to these quantitative differences, Jane produced a number of atypical consonant substitutions (such as, d/b, d/f, j/l, j/r/, w/t), which was a noted red flag. Based on these results, Jane presents both qualitative and quantitative differences from what would be expected at this age. Therefore, she is considered to present a deviant pattern in her phonological development. In addition to recommendations to the parents for ways to stimulate and facilitate Jane's phonological and lexical development, enrollment in early intervention to increase her phonetic inventory, word structure, and vocabulary is recommended.

CASE STUDY: JOEY, AGE 24 MONTHS

Joey, a child with typical speech and language development, was raised in a two-parent home where GAE was spoken. His phonological skills were assessed as part of the PEEPS project described above. A summary of findings for Joey is presented below, and a full transcript and analysis of his productions are shown in Appendix 5.3.

Number of Words Produced

Joey produced 49 of the 60 words in the PEEPS Word List. Of these, 29 were produced spontaneously and 20 were imitations.

Independent Analysis

Findings from the independent analysis of Joey's speech productions were as follows.

Phonetic Inventory   In word-initial position, Joey produced 11 different singleton consonants and two consonant clusters. His repertoire included 5 stops [p, b, t, d, k], 2 fricatives [f, s], 2 nasals [m, n], and 2 glides [w, h]. Taken together, he had 4 different manner classes and 5 places of articulation. He also produced 2 clusters: [tw-] and [bw-] (which is not a cluster in adult English).

In word-final position, Joey's inventory included 9 consonants and 2 consonant clusters. His consonantal repertoire included stops [p, t, d, k], fricatives [f, s, z], and nasals [m, n]. In addition, he produced an alveolar affricate [ts] in his production of *watch* [wats]; this phone is not a phoneme of English. Joey produced 2 consonant clusters [-nt, -ŋk]. In total, Joey had 10 different singleton consonants—4 manner classes and 4 places of articulation.

Word and Syllable Shapes   Joey's syllable structures included monosyllabic and disyllabic forms: CV, CVC, CVCV, CVCVC, as well as initial and final clusters: CC-, -CC, and two words with a consonant sequence: -VCCV- in his pronunciation of *monkey, blanket,* and *finger.*

Summary of Independent Analysis

- 11 word-initial consonants and 2 consonant clusters

- 9 word-final consonants and 2 clusters

- Places of articulation: labial, labiodental, alveolar, palatal, glottal

- Manner of articulation: stop, fricative, affricate, nasal, glide

- Word-initial phonetic inventory is larger than word-final phonetic inventory

- Syllable structures: mono- and disyllabic productions; initial and final consonant clusters

Relational Analysis

Findings from the relational analysis of Joey's speech productions were as follows.

Error Patterns   Word-initially, Joey produced stops for target fricatives and affricates; he also reduced consonant clusters. Word-finally, Joey's most common errors involved deletions. Errors affecting word and syllable structure include syllable omission in *elephant* and *banana*, and addition of schwa in the imitated production of *bug* (yielding [bʌɡə] and *bib* [bɪbə]).

Accuracy: PCC = 74.5% accuracy

WS Match: 67.3% match

Summary of Relational Analysis

Joey's profile is within the expectations outlined in the PEEPS 24-month Profile for all measures. See Table 5.4 in the section "Age-Level Profiles."

Comparison to PEEPS Profile and Clinical Impression

The phonological analysis of Joey's productions was compared to the PEEPS Profile at 24 months (see Table 6.1). The comparison is summarized in Table 5.3. below.

AGE-LEVEL PROFILES

The following sections provide an overview of speech and language development in children 18–36 months and a set of age-related profiles for phonetic and phonological acquisition. Specifically, the age-level profiles will include the following ages:

- 18–21 months
- 24 months
- 27–30 months
- 33–36 months

Table 5.3.   Comparison of Joey's phonological analysis to 24-month PEEPS Profile

	Joey's Analysis (age 24 months)	PEEPS Profile: 24 months
Vocabulary	Within normal range	
PEEPS words produced	49 words	49.5
Phonetic Inventory		
Word-initial consonants	11 singleton Cs 2 consonant clusters	13.6 2.5
Word-final consonants	9 singleton Cs 2 consonant clusters	11.6 1.9
Manner classes	4 classes word-initial: stop, fricative, nasal, glide 4 classes word-final: stop, fricative, affricate, nasal	Table 6.1 includes all classes
Places of articulation	6 places word-initial: labial, labiodental, alveolar, palatal velar, glottal 4 places word-final: stop, fricative, affricate, nasal	Table 6.1 includes all classes
Word and syllable shapes	Mono- and disyllables Final consonants Initial and final clusters	
Relational analysis **PCC** **WSM**	74.5% 67.3%	71.3% 68.2%

It is important to note that measures of children's speech and language abilities are likely to vary from one study to another due to differences in data collection and data analysis. For example, measures taken from *conversational speech samples* will likely differ from those based on *assessment tests* wherein the word list is fixed and may include words and phonetic elements that are beyond the child's abilities. In conversational interactions, children choose the words they wish to produce and, consequently, speech output may be more accurate because the words are phonologically easier. For children ages 18–24 months, the words may include a reduced range of phonetic elements and word shapes. In contrast, children ages 33–36 months may produce longer and more utterances, and in these cases, intelligibility is often reduced.

Productions gathered through formal assessment tests, using a specific list of words, may include items that are not in the child's active vocabulary. Consequently, some words may not be produced at all, or may be elicited as imitated responses. Both approaches to data collection (conversational speech and assessment tests) are valuable and provide important insights into a child's developing phonological system. At the same time, we should recognize that the outcome measures may be different. This is the value of PEEPS that includes age-appropriate vocabulary with representative phonetic features.

The sections below summarize data on phonological acquisition in children 18–36 months, incorporating, where possible, data from a variety of studies. The general expectations for language development provided below include:

- Size of productive vocabulary
- Intelligibility (proportion of speech that can be understood by an individual not familiar with child's speech)
- Mean length of utterance in words.

Expectations for phonetic and phonological systems include those measures assessed by PEEPS:

- Consonantal inventories
- Phonetic feature classes of consonants in the word-initial and word-final inventories
- The types of syllable and word shapes produced
- The accuracy of word shapes
- Percentage of Consonants Correct (PCC) for the entire sample

These profiles are based on large-scale studies and on findings from PEEPS assessments at four age levels: (a) 18–21 months, (b) 24 months, (c) 27–30 months, (d) 33–36 months (Crowe & McLeod, 2020; Smit, 1986; Smit et al., 1990; Stoel-Gammon, 1985; 1987).

PEEPS Profile: Age 18–21 Months

Table 5.4 shows the PEEPS Profile for a typically developing child at age 18–21 months.

PEEPS Profile: Age 24 Months

Table 5.4 shows the PEEPS Profile for a typically developing child at age 24 months.

PEEPS Profile: Age 27–30 Months

Table 5.5 shows the PEEPS Profile for a typically developing child at age 27–30 months.

PEEPS Profile: Age 33–36 Months

Table 5.6 shows the PEEPS Profile for a typically developing child at age 33–36 months.

See Appendix C at the end of the book for a comprehensive summary of expected overall language, phonological, physical, and cognitive development from birth to age 6.

Table 5.4. PEEPS Profile: 18–21 months

Language	Phonetic and Phonological Development

Lexicon size
• At 18 months, the typical child is in the "first-word stage" with an expressive vocabulary of about 50 words.
• By 21 months, vocabulary size has increased to about 125 words with considerable variation.
  • There is a great deal of individual variation in vocabulary size and many utterances during this period are unintelligible.
 	
Intelligibility
• During the period of 18–21 months, intelligibility of children's speech is low, reported to be less than 50%, with great individual variation (Flipsen, Jr., 2006).
 	
Length of utterance in words
• One to two words
	Findings from spontaneous speech samples (Stoel-Gammon, 1985)
	• Mean # different initial Cs: 6.3
	• Mean # different final Cs: 2.8
	• Manner classes: stop, nasal, glide
	• Places of articulation: labial; alveolar (velar, glottal)
	
	Findings from PEEPS assessments
	• Mean number of PEEPS words produced:
	  • 18m: 22.6 words
	  • 21m: 27.9 words
	• Mean # different **Initial Consonants**:
	  • 18m: 9.6 consonants
	  • 21m: 11.0 consonants
	• Mean # different **Final Consonants**:
	  • 18m: 3.8 consonants
	  • 21m: 6.7 consonants
	• Manner classes:
	  • Stop
	  • Nasal
	  • Glide
	• Places of articulation:
	  • Labial
	  • Labiodental
	  • Alveolar
	  • Emerging: velar, glottal
	• Word and syllable shapes
	  • Word shapes - Number of syllables:
	    • 85%–87% of children produced words of 1 and 2 syllables.
	    • No children produced 3-syllable words.
	• Mean # different clusters:
	  • 18m: 0
	  • 21m: 0.6 initial position; 0.3 final position
	• Accuracy of word shapes (*PEEPS*):
	  • 18m: 41.3%
	  • 21m: 48.4%
	• Consonantal Accuracy: PEEPS
	  • Percent Consonants Correct:
	    • 18m: 47.5%
	    • 21m: 58.3%

Key: C, consonants; m, months.

Warning Signs of Impairment at 2 Years

As noted in Chapter 4, red flags for phonetic and phonological development include numerous vowel errors, frequent deletion of initial consonants, frequent use of glottal stop or [h] for a variety of consonants, backing (e.g., [ku] for "two"), and, final consonant deletion, particularly as the child approaches 3 years (Stoel-Gammon, 1987).

Williams and Elbert (2003) reported that predictors of LTs' phonological skills include both quantitative and qualitative characteristics. Specifically, at age 2 years, 9 months,

Table 5.5. PEEPS Profile: 27–30 months

Language	Phonetic and Phonological Development

Lexicon size
• At age 27–30 months, vocabulary size is 450–550 words, with great individual variation.
 	
Intelligibility
• 70%–75% (Flipsen, Jr., 2006)
 	
Length of utterance in words
• Multi-word sentences
	Findings from PEEPS assessments
	• Mean # number of PEEPS words produced:
	  • 27m: 49.5 words
	  • 30m: 51.7 words
	• Mean # different **Initial Consonants**:
	  • 27m: 14.1 consonants
	  • 30m: 15.0 consonants
	• Mean # different **Final Consonants**:
	  • 27m: 10.7 consonants
	  • 30m: 13.9 consonants
	• Manner classes:
	  • Stop
	  • Nasal
	  • Glide
	  • Fricative
	  • Affricate
	  • Liquid
	• Places of articulation:
	  • Labial
	  • Labiodental
	  • Alveolar
	  • Palatal
	  • Velar
	  • Glottal
	  • Emerging: interdental
	Word and syllable shapes
	• Word shapes: Number of syllables
	  • All children produced words of 1 and 2 syllables.
	  • 50%–60% of children produced 3-syllable words.
	• Consonant clusters:
	  • mean # different clusters:
	    • **Initial** position:
	      • 27m: 3.2 clusters
	      • 30m: 3.6 clusters
	    • **Final** position:
	      • 27m: 1.6 clusters
	      • 30m: 2.5 clusters
	  • PEEPS: Accuracy of word shapes:
	    • 27m: 65.9%
	    • 30m: 83.4%
	Consonantal Accuracy (PCC):
	PEEPS (elicited words):
	  • 27m: 65.1% (range 43%–88%)
	  • 30m: 83.7% (range 70%–93%)

Key: m, months.

children who present with the following cluster of phonological/phonetic characteristics are less likely to demonstrate spontaneous recovery and catch up with their age peers without direct intervention. This cluster of characteristics includes smaller phonetic inventories, simple and less diverse syllable structures, lower PCC scores, greater sound variability, and atypical error patterns.

Table 5.6.   PEEPS Profile: 33–36 months

Language	Phonetic and Phonological Development
Lexicon size	**Findings from PEEPS assessments**

• At age 33–36 months, vocabulary size is typically > 1,000 words, with great individual variation.	• Mean # number of PEEPS words produced:
	  • 33m: 54.1 words
	  • 36m: 56.1 words
	  • Note: On average, nearly all *PEEPS* words were produced.

Intelligibility	• Mean # different **Initial Consonants**:
	  • 33m: 15.0 consonants
	  • 36m: 15.5 consonants

• 70%–90% (great individual variation; Flipsen, Jr., 2006)	• Mean # different **Final Consonants**:
	  • 33m: 12.1 consonants
	  • 36m: 15.7 consonants

Length of utterance in words	• Manner classes:
	  • Stop
	  • Nasal
	  • Glide
	  • Fricative
	  • Affricate
	  • Liquid

• Multi-word sentences	• Places of articulation:
	  • Labial
	  • Labiodental
	  • Alveolar
	  • Palatal
	  • Velar
	  • Glottal
	  • Emerging: interdental

	Word and syllable shapes
	• Word shapes: Number of syllables
	  • All children produced mono- and di-syllables.
	  • 50%–60% of children produced 3-syllable words,
	• Consonant clusters:
	  • mean # different clusters:
	    • **Initial** position:
	      • 33m: 3.9 clusters
	      • 36m: 4.9 clusters
	    • **Final** position:
	      • 27m: 2.5 clusters
	      • 30m: 3.2 clusters
	• PEEPS: Accuracy of word shapes:
	  • 33m: 75.6%
	  • 36m: 87.6%

	Consonantal Accuracy (PCC):
	PEEPS (elicited words):
	  • 33m: 76.7%
	  • 36m: 83.3%
	Note: the high number for PCC is, in part, a result of the word selection criteria for PEEPS. Remember that the main criterion for words is *age of acquisition* and most early acquired words have early acquired consonants.

Key: m, months.

SUMMARY

Case studies of three children of different ages and phonological abilities were presented from a PEEPS analysis. Each child's independent and relational analyses was compared to the appropriate Developmental Profile to determine if the child's phonological skills were delayed, deviant, or typical. Developmental Profiles were provided for each of the following ages: 18–21 months; 24 months; 27–30 months; and 33–36 months. These profiles are used by clinicians to interpret a child's phonological development. Finally, the cluster of qualitative and quantitative warning signs for impairment at age 2 was summarized. In Chapter 6, data are summarized from children who exhibited typical phonological development from ages 18 to 36 months.

Sample Completed PEEPS Analysis Form: Nick

The following pages show a sample completed PEEPS form for Nick, a 22-month-old boy.

PEEPS Summary Analysis and Word List

Child's name: *Nick*	Test age *(months)*: *22*	# Words Produced:	
Date of birth *(Y/M/D)*: *2020/10/9*	Gender: *male*		*NOTES*
Date tested *(Y/M/D)*: *2022/8/15*	Examiner: *ALW*	*22 / 60*	*He produced "ball" and "woof" 2x each.*

Independent Analysis

Circle consonants and consonant clusters produced in each word position. Add consonants and clusters produced but not listed.

Consonant Inventory

Word-Initial Consonants	p	(b)	(t)	(d)	k	g	s	f	s	z	(ʃ)	tʃ	dʒ	(m)	(n)	l	ɹ	(w)	h	Other: *n/a*	Total: 7

Word-Initial Clusters	bl-	tɹ-	dʒ-	kw-	sp-	st-														Other: *n/a*	Total: 0

Word-Initial Manner	(Stop)		(Fricative)		Affricate		(Nasal)			Liquid		Glide		# Manner Classes: 4

Word-Initial Place	(Labial/labiodental)		Alveolar/interdental		(Palatal)		Velar		Glottal		# Places: 3

Word-Final Consonants	p	b	t	d	k	g	θ	f	(s)	z	ʃ	tʃ	m	n	ŋ	l	(ɹ)			Other: *?*	Total: 3

Word-Final Clusters	-nd	-ŋk	-nt																	Other: *-ps*	Total: 1

Word-Final Manner	(Stop)		(Fricative)		Affricate		(Nasal)			(Liquid)				# Manner Classes: 3

Word-Final Place	Labial/labiodental		Alveolar/interdental		(Palatal)		(Velar)				# Places: 3

Word and Syllable Shapes: Circle those that occur.

Presence of: (Final consonant(s)) Initial consonant(s) (Final consonant cluster)

Number of syllables: (1) (2) 3

Relational Analysis

	Accuracy		
# WS Match / # Words Produced:	*13 / 22*	**WSM:** *59.1%*	
PCC Child / PCC Target:	*15 / 40*	**PCC:** *37.5%*	

Number of Syllables	
2-syllable	(Y) / N
3-syllable	Y / (N)

Red Flags (See Manual for examples.)	
WF inventory substantially > WI inventory	Y / (N)
Unusual Vowel Errors	Y / (N)
Atypical Consonant Substitutions	Y / (N)
Atypical Deletions	Y / (N)

APPENDIX 5.1 *(continued)*

Word	IPA: Target	IPA: Child	WS Target	WSM	Initial C: Target	Initial C: Child	Final C: Target	Final C: Child	S/I	PCC: Child	PCC: Target	Notes
cow	kaʊ	daʊ	CV	1	k	d			S	0	1	
moo	mu	mu	CV	1	m	m			S	1	1	
dog	dɑg	dɑ	CVC	0	d	d	g	—	S	1	2	
woof	wʊf	wʊ	CVC	0	w	w	f	—	S	1	2	Said "woof" 2x, 2nd time as /ɹʊ/
duck(y)	dʌk(i)	dʌʔ	CVC(V)	1	d	d	(k)	ʔ	S	1	2	
quack	kwæk	NR	CCVC	NR	kw	NR	k	NR	NR	NR	~~3~~	
fish(y)	fɪʃ(i)	NR	CVC(V)	NR	f	NR	(ʃ)	NR	NR	NR	~~2~~	
bird	bɝd	bɝ	CVC	0	b	b	d	—	S	1	2	
kitty (cat)	kɪt/di (kæt)	NR	CVCV(CVC)	NR	k	NR	(t)	NR	NR	NR	~~2(4)~~	
puppy	pʌpi	NR	CVCV	NR	p	NR	p	NR	NR	NR	~~2~~	
*mouse	maʊs	NR	CVC	NR	m	NR	s	NR	NR	NR	~~2~~	
pig(gy)	pɪg(i)	bɪ	CVC(V)	0	p	b	(g)	—	S	0	2	
*sheep	ʃip	NR	CVC	NR	ʃ	NR	p	NR	NR	NR	~~2~~	
chicken	tʃɪkən	NR	CVCVC	NR	tʃ	NR	n	NR	NR	NR	~~3~~	
bug	bʌg	NR	CVC	NR	b	NR	g	NR	NR	NR	~~2~~	
*elephant	ɛləfənt	NR	VCVCVCC	NR			nt	NR	NR	NR	~~4~~	
*monkey	mʌŋki	NR	CVCCV	NR	m	NR		NR	NR	NR	~~3~~	
*lion	laɪ(j)ən	NR	CV(C)VC	NR	l	NR	n	NR	NR	NR	~~2(3)~~	
baby	beɪbi	beɪbi	CVCV	1	b	b			S	2	2	
ear	ɹɪ	ɹɪ	VC	1			ɹ	ɹ	S	1	1	
# words produced by child/# words possible	9 / 20		# match	5/9					Total PCC	8	15	

APPENDIX 5.1 *(continued)*

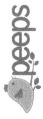peeps

Word	IPA: Target	IPA: Child	WS Target	WSM	Initial C: Target	Initial C: Child	Final C: Target	Final C: Child	S/I	PCC: Child	PCC: Target	Notes
finger	fɪŋgɚ	NR	CVCCV	NR	f	NR			NR	NR	~~3~~	
*foot	fʊt	dʊʔ	CVC	1	f	d	t	ʔ	S	0	2	
hair	hɛɹ	NR	CVC	NR	h	NR	ɹ	NR	NR	NR	~~2~~	
hand	hænd	NR	CVCC	NR	h	NR	nd	NR	NR	NR	~~3~~	
mouth	maʊθ	maʊʔ	CVC	1	m	m	θ	ʔ	S	1	2	
nose	noʊz	noʊ	CVC	0	n	n	z	--	S	1	2	
toe(s)	toʊ(z)	toʊ	CV(C)	1	t	t	(z)	--	S	1	1/~~2~~	
*tummy	tʌmi	NR	CVCV	NR	t	NR		NR	NR	NR	~~2~~	
*tongue	tʌŋ	NR	CVC	NR	t	NR	ŋ	NR	NR	NR	~~2~~	
belly button	bɛlibʌtən	NR	CVCVCVC	NR	b	NR	n	NR	NR	NR	~~5~~	
*soap	soʊp	NR	CVC	NR	s	NR	p	NR	NR	NR	~~2~~	
*comb	koʊm	NR	CVC	NR	k	NR	m	NR	NR	NR	~~2~~	
blanket	blæŋkət	NR	CCVCCVC	NR	bl	NR	t	NR	NR	NR	~~5~~	
peek-a-boo	pikabu	NR	CVCVCV	NR	p	NR			NR	NR	~~3~~	
*doll	dɑl	NR	CVC	NR	d	NR	l	NR	NR	NR	~~2~~	
shoe	ʃu	ʃu	CV	1	ʃ	ʃ			S	1	1	
*sock	sɑk	NR	CVC	NR	s	NR	k	NR	NR	NR	~~2~~	
*zipper	zɪpɚ	NR	CVCV	NR	z	NR		NR	NR	NR	~~2~~	
hat	hæt	æʔ	CVC	0	h	--	t	ʔ	S	0	2	
off	ɑf	NR	VC	NR			f	NR	NR	NR	~~1~~	
# words produced by child/# words possible	6/20		# match	4/6					Total PCC	4	10	

*indicates words acquired between 22–24 months

74

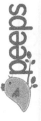
peeps

Word	IPA: Target	IPA: Child	WS Target	WSM	Initial C: Target	Initial C: Child	Final C: Target	Final C: Child	S/I	PCC: Child	PCC: Target	Notes
diaper	daɪpɚ	NR	CVCV	NR	d	NR			NR	NR	~~2~~	
*bib	bɪb	NR	CVC	NR	b	NR	b	NR	NR	NR	~~2~~	
juice	ʤus	dus	CVC	1	ʤ	d	s	s	S	1	2	
banana	bənænə	NR	CVCVCV	NR	b	NR			NR	NR	~~3~~	
cookie	kʊki	NR	CVCV	NR	k	NR			NR	NR	~~2~~	
cheese	ʧiz	dis	CVC	1	ʧ	d	z	s	S	0	2	
cup	kʌp	ʌʔ	CVC	0	k	–	p	ʔ	S	0	2	
drink	dɹɪŋk	NR	CCVCC	NR	dɹ	NR	ŋk	NR	NR	NR	~~4~~	
bottle	bɑt/dəl	NR	CVCVC	NR	b	NR	l	NR	NR	NR	~~3~~	
spoon	spun	NR	CCVC	NR	sp	NR	n	NR	NR	NR	~~3~~	
*train	tɹeɪn	NR	CCVC	NR	tɹ	NR	n	NR	NR	NR	~~3~~	
truck	tɹʌk	dʌʔ	CCVC	0	tɹ	d	k	ʔ	1	0	3	
*stop	stɑp	NR	CCVC	NR	st	NR	p	NR	NR	NR	~~3~~	
go	goʊ	doʊ	CV	1	g	d			S	0	1	
light	laɪt	NR	CVC	NR	l	NR	t	NR	NR	NR	~~2~~	
balloon	bəlun	NR	CVCVC	NR	b	NR	n	NR	NR	NR	~~3~~	
ball	bɑl	bɑʔ	CVC	1	b	b	l	ʔ	S	1	2	*Said "ball" 2x, 2nd time as /bɑ/*
*rock	ɹɑk	NR	CVC	NR	ɹ	NR	k	NR	NR	NR	~~2~~	
*block	blɑk	wɑps	CCVC	0	bl	w	k	ps	S	0	3	
*watch	wɑʧ	NR	CVC	NR	w	NR	ʧ	NR	NR	NR	~~2~~	
# words produced by child/# words possible	7/20		# match	4/7					Total PCC	3	15	

*indicates words acquired between 22–24 months

Sample Completed PEEPS Analysis Form: Jane

The following pages show a sample completed PEEPS form for Jane, a 32-month-old girl.

PEEPS Summary Analysis and Word List

Child's name: Jane	Test age (months): 32	NOTES	# Words Produced:	Atypical consonant substitutions: d/b, j/kw, d/f, j/l, w/t
Date of birth (Y/M/D): 2019/11/8	Gender: female			
Date tested (Y/M/D): 2022/8/15	Examiner: ALW		29 / 60	

Independent Analysis

Circle consonants and consonant clusters produced in each word position. Add consonants and clusters produced but not listed.

Consonant Inventory

Word-Initial Consonants	p	b	t	(d)	k	g	f	s	z	ʃ	tʃ	(dʒ)	(m)	(n)	ɹ	(w)	(h)	**Other:** j	**Total:** 7
Word-Initial Clusters	bl-	tɹ-	dɹ-	kw-	sp-	st-												**Other:** n/a	**Total:** 0
Word-Initial Manner	(Stop)			Fricative			Affricate			(Nasal)			Liquid			(Glide)		**# Manner Classes:** 3
Word-Initial Place	(Labial/labiodental)			(Alveolar/interdental)						(Palatal)			Velar			(Glottal)		**# Places:** 4
Word-Final Consonants	p	b	t	d	k	g	f	θ	s	z	ʃ	tʃ	m	n	ŋ	l	ɹ	**Other:** n/a	**Total:** 0
Word-Final Clusters	-nd	-nt	-ŋk															**Other:** n/a	**Total:** 0
Word-Final Manner	Stop						Fricative					Affricate	Nasal			Liquid		**# Manner Classes:** 0
Word-Final Place	Labial/labiodental						Alveolar/interdental					Palatal				Velar		**# Places:** 0

Word and Syllable Shapes: Circle those that occur.

Presence of: Final consonant(s) Initial consonant cluster Final consonant cluster

Number of syllables: (1) (2) 3

Number of Syllables		
2-syllable	(Y) / N	
3-syllable	Y / (N)	

Relational Analysis

	Accuracy		
# WS Match / # Words Produced:	8 / 29	WSM: 27.6%	
PCC Child / PCC Target:	10 / 56	PCC: 17.8%	

Red Flags (See Manual for examples.)	
WF inventory substantially > WI inventory	Y / (N)
Unusual Vowel Errors	Y / (N)
Atypical Consonant Substitutions	(Y) / N
Atypical Deletions	Y / (N)

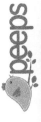

Word	IPA: Target	IPA: Child	WS Target	WSM	Initial C: Target	Initial C: Child	Final C: Target	Final C: Child	S/I	PCC: Child	PCC: Target	Notes
cow	kaʊ	daʊ	CV	1	k	d			S	0	1	
moo	mu	mu	CV	1	m	m			S	1	1	
dog	dɑg	dɑ	CVC	0	d	d	g	--	S	1	2	
woof	wʊf	NR	CVC	NR	w	NR	f	NR	NR	NR	~~2~~	
duck(y)	dʌk(i)	dʌ	CVC(V)	0	d	d	(k)	0	S	1	2	
quack	kwæk	æ	CCVC	0	kw	--	k	--	S	0	3	
fish(y)	fɪʃ(i)	dɪ	CVC(V)	0	f	d	(ʃ)	--	S	0	2	
bird	bɚd	NR	CVC	NR	b	NR	d	NR	NR	NR	~~2~~	
kitty (cat)	kɪti/di (kæt)	NR	CVCV(CVC)	NR	k	NR	(t)	NR	NR	NR	~~2(4)~~	
puppy	pʌpi	NR	CVCV	NR	p	NR			NR	NR	~~2~~	
*mouse	maʊs	maʊ	CVC	0	m	m	s	--	S	1	2	
pig(gy)	pɪg(i)	dɪ	CVC(V)	0	p	d	(g)	--	S	0	2	
*sheep	ʃip	NR	CVC	NR	ʃ	NR	p	NR	NR	NR	~~2~~	
chicken	tʃɪkən	NR	CVCVC	NR	tʃ	NR	n	NR	NR	NR	~~3~~	
bug	bʌg	NR	CVC	NR	b	NR	g	NR	NR	NR	~~2~~	
*elephant	ɛləfənt	NR	VCVCVCC	NR			nt	NR	NR	NR	~~4~~	
*monkey	mʌŋki	NR	CVCCV	NR	m	NR			NR	NR	~~3~~	
*lion	laɪ(j)ən	NR	CVI(C)VC	NR	l	NR	n	NR	NR	NR	~~2(3)~~	
baby	beɪbi	deɪdi	CVCV	1	b	d			S	0	2	
ear	ɪɹ	NR	VC	NR			ɹ	NR	NR	NR	~~1~~	
# words produced by child / # words possible	9/20		# match	3/9				Total PCC		4	17	

*indicates words acquired between 22–24 months

(continued)

77

APPENDIX 5.2 *(continued)*

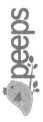

Word	IPA: Target	IPA: Child	WS Target	WSM	Initial C: Target	Initial C: Child	Final C: Target	Final C: Child	S/I	PCC: Child	PCC: Target	Notes
finger	fɪŋɡɚ	NR	CVCCV	NR	f	NR			NR	NR	3̶	
*foot	fʊt	dʊ	CVC	0	f	d	t	--	S	0	2	
hair	hɛɹ	hɛ	CVC	0	h	h	ɹ	--	S	1	2	
hand	hænd	NR	CVCC	NR	h	NR	nd	NR	NR	NR	3̶	
mouth	maʊθ	maʊ	CVC	0	m	m	θ	--	S	1	2	
nose	noʊz	noʊ	CVC	0	n	n	z	--	S	1	2	
toe(s)	toʊ(z)	doʊ	CV(C)	1	t	d	(z)	--	S	0	1̶(2̶)	Said "toe" 2x, 2nd time as /woʊ/
*tummy	tʌmi	dʌmi	CVCV	1	t	d			m	1	2	
*tongue	tʌŋ	NR	CVC	NR	t	NR	ŋ	NR	NR	NR	2̶	
belly button	bɛlibʌtən	NR	CVCVCVC	NR	b	NR	n	NR	NR	NR	5̶	
*soap	soʊp	NR	CVC	NR	s	NR	p	NR	NR	NR	2̶	
*comb	koʊm	NR	CVC	NR	k	NR	m	NR	NR	NR	2̶	
blanket	blæŋkɛt	NR	CCVCCVC	NR	bl	NR	t	NR	NR	NR	5̶	
peek-a-boo	pikabu	mimu	CVCVCV	0	p	m		NR	S	0	3	
*doll	dɑl	dɑ	CVC	0	d	d	l	--	S	1	2	
shoe	ʃu	du	CV	1	ʃ	d			S	0	1	
*sock	sɑk	dɑ	CVC	0	s	d	k	--	S	0	2	
*zipper	zɪpɚ	NR	CVCV	NR	z	NR			NR	NR	2̶	
hat	hæt	hæ	CVC	0	h	h	t	--	S	1	2	
off	ɑf	NR	VC	NR			f	NR	NR	NR	1̶	
# words produced by child/# words possible	11/20		# match	3/11						Total PCC		
										6	21	

*indicates words acquired between 22–24 months

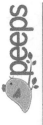

Word	IPA: Target	IPA: Child	WS Target	WSM	Initial C: Target	Initial C: Child	Final C: Target	Final C: Child	S/I	PCC: Child	PCC: Target	Notes
diaper	daɪpɚ	NR	CVCV	NR	d	NR			NR	NR	~~2~~	
*bib	bɪb	NR	CVC	NR	b	NR	b	NR	NR	NR	~~2~~	
juice	dʒus	du	CVC	0	dʒ	d	s	--	S	0	2	
banana	bənænə	NR	CVCVCV	NR	b	NR			NR	NR	~~3~~	
cookie	kʊki	dʊdi	CVCV	1	k	d			S	0	2	
cheese	tʃiz	di	CVC	0	tʃ	d	z	--	S	0	2	
cup	kʌp	dʌ	CVC	0	k	d	p	--	S	0	2	
drink	dɹɪŋk	NR	CCVCC	NR	dɹ	NR	ŋk	NR	NR	NR	~~4~~	
bottle	bɑt/bɑl	NR	CVCVC	NR	b	NR	l	NR	NR	NR	~~3~~	
spoon	spun	NR	CCVC	NR	sp	NR	n	NR	NR	NR	~~3~~	
*train	tɹeɪn	NR	CCVC	NR	tɹ	NR	n	NR	NR	NR	~~3~~	
truck	tɹʌk	dʌ	CCVC	0	tɹ	d	k	--	S	0	3	
*stop	stɑp	NR	CCVC	NR	st	NR	p	NR	NR	NR	~~3~~	
go	goʊ	doʊ	CV	1	g	d			S	0	1	
light	laɪt	dʒaɪ	CVC	0	l	dʒ	t	--	S	0	2	
balloon	bəlun	NR	CVCVC	NR	b	NR	n	NR	NR	NR	~~3~~	
ball	bɑl	dɑ	CVC	0	b	d	l	--	S	0	2	
*rock	ɹɑk	dʒɑ	CVC	0	ɹ	dʒ	k	--	S	0	2	
*block	blɑk	NR	CCVC	NR	bl	NR	k	NR	NR	NR	~~3~~	
*watch	wɑtʃ	NR	CVC	NR	w	NR	tʃ	NR	NR	NR	~~2~~	
# words produced by child/# words possible		9/20	# match	2/9					Total PCC	0	18	

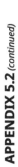

Sample Completed PEEPS Analysis Form: Joey

The following pages show a sample completed PEEPS form for Joey, a 24-month-old boy.

PEEPS Summary Analysis and Word List

Child's name: Joey	Test age (months): 24	# Words Produced:
Date of birth (Y/M/D): 2020/7/1	Gender: male	
Date tested (Y/M/D): 2022/7/1	Examiner: CSG	49 / 60

NOTES

Independent Analysis

Circle consonants and consonant clusters produced in each word position. Add consonants and clusters produced but not listed.

Consonant Inventory

Word-Initial Consonants	(p)	(b)	(t)	(d)	(k)	g	(f)	(s)	z	ʃ	tʃ	dʒ	(m)	(n)	l	ɹ	(w)	(h)		Other: n/a	Total: 11
Word-Initial Clusters	bl-	tɹ-	dʒ-	kw-	sp-	st-														Other: bw-, tw-	Total: 2
Word-Initial Manner	(Stop)		(Fricative)				(Affricate)				(Nasal)		(Liquid)				(Glide)			# Manner Classes: 4	
Word-Initial Place	(Labial) (Labiodental)						(Alveolar) (Interdental)				(Palatal)		(Velar)				(Glottal)			# Places: 6	
Word-Final Consonants	(p)	b	(t)	d	(k)	g	(f)	(s)	(z)	ʃ	tʃ		(m)	(n)	(ŋ)	ɹ				Other: ts	Total: 9
Word-Final Clusters	-nt	-ŋk	-nd																	Other: n/a	Total: 2
Word-Final Manner			(Stop)				(Fricative)				(Affricate)		(Nasal)				(Liquid)			# Manner Classes: 4	
Word-Final Place			(Labial) (Labiodental)				(Alveolar) (Interdental)				Palatal		(Velar)							# Places: 4	

Word and Syllable Shapes: Circle those that occur.

Presence of: (Final consonant(s)) (Initial consonant cluster) (Final consonant cluster)

Number of syllables: (1) (2) 3

Relational Analysis

Accuracy			
# WS Match / # Words Produced:	33 / 49	WSM:	67.3%
PCC Child / PCC Target:	82 / 110	PCC:	74.5%

Number of Syllables	
2-syllable	(Y) / N
3-syllable	Y / (N)

Red Flags (See Manual for examples.)	
WF inventory substantially > WI inventory	Y / (N)
Unusual Vowel Errors	Y / (N)
Atypical Consonant Substitutions	Y / (N)
Atypical Deletions	Y / (N)

Word	IPA: Target	IPA: Child	WS Target	WSM	Initial C: Target	Initial C: Child	Final C: Target	Final C: Child	S/I	PCC: Child	PCC: Target	Notes
cow	kaʊ	kaʊ	CV	1	k	k			S	1	1	
moo	mu	mu	CV	1	m	m			S	1	1	
dog	dɑg	da	CVC	0	d	d	g	--	S	1	2	
woof	wʊf	wʊf	CVC	1	w	w	f	f	1	2	2	
duck(y)	dʌk(i)	dʌki	CVC(V)	1	d	d	(k)	f	S	2	2	CVCV structure
quack	kwæk	NR	CCVC	NR	kw	NR	k	NR	NR	NR	3̶	
fish(y)	fɪʃ(i)	fɪs	CVC(V)	1	f	f	(ʃ)	s	S	1	2	
bird	bɝd	bɔd	CVC	1	b	b	d	d	S	2	2	
kitty (cat)	kɪt/di (kæt)	kæt	CVCV(CVC)	1	k	k	(t)	t	S	2	2(4̶)	
puppy	pʌpi	pʌpi	CVCV	1	p	p			S	2	2	
*mouse	maʊs	maʊs	CVC	1	m	m	s	s	S	2	2	
pig(gy)	pɪg(i)	pɪgə	CVC(V)	0	p	p	(g)	schwa	1	2	2	schwa added
*sheep	ʃip	sip	CVC	1	ʃ	s	p	p	S	1	2	
chicken	tʃɪkən	tɪkən	CVCVC	1	tʃ	t	n	n	S	2	3	
bug	bʌg	bʌgə	CVC	0	b	b	g	schwa	1	2	2	schwa added
*elephant	ɛləfənt	ɛfʌnt	VCVCVCC	0			nt	nt	1	3	4	
*monkey	mʌŋki	mʌŋki	CVCCV	1	m	m			1	3	3	
*lion	laɪ(j)ən	laɪən	CV(C)VC	1	l	ɹ	n	n	1	2	2(3̶)	
baby	beɪbi	beɪbi	CVCV	1	b	b			S	2	2	
ear	ɪɹ	eɪ	VC	0			ɹ	schwa	S	0	1	Vowelization
# words produced by child/# words possible	19/20		# match	14/19					Total PCC	33	39	

*indicates words acquired between 22–24 months

(continued)

APPENDIX 5.3 *(continued)*

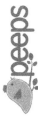

Word	IPA: Target	IPA: Child	WS Target	WSM	Initial C: Target	Initial C: Child	Final C: Target	Final C: Child	S/I	PCC: Child	PCC: Target	Notes
finger	frŋgɚ	NR	CVCCV	NR	f	NR			NR	NR	~~3~~	
*foot	fʊt	NR	CVC	NR	f	NR	t	NR	NR	NR	~~2~~	
hair	hɛɹ	hɛə	CVC	0	h	h	ɹ	schwa	S	1	2	vowelization
hand	hænd	NR	CVCC	NR	h	NR	nd	NR	NR	NR	~~3~~	
mouth	maʊθ	maʊf	CVC	1	m	m	θ	f	S	1	2	
nose	noʊz	noʊz	CVC	1	n	n	z	z	S	2	2	
toe(s)	toʊ(z)	toʊz	CV(C)	1	t	t	(z)	z	1	2	~~1~~(2)	
*tummy	tʌmi	tʌmi	CVCV	1	t	t			S	2	2	
*tongue	tʌŋ	NR	CVC	NR	t	NR	ŋ	NR	NR	NR	~~2~~	
belly button	bɛlibʌtən	bʌtɪn	CVCVCVCVC	0	b	b	n	n	1	3	5	
*soap	soʊp	soʊp	CVC	1	s	s	p	p	1	2	2	
*comb	koʊm	koʊm	CVC	1	k	k	m	m	1	2	2	
blanket	blæŋkət	bæŋki	CCVCCVC	0	bl	b	t	--	S	3	5	
peek-a-boo	pikabu	NR	CVCVCV	NR	p	NR			NR	NR	~~3~~	
*doll	dɑl	dɑ	CVC	0	d	d	l	--	S	1	2	
shoe	ʃu	ʃu	CV	1	ʃ	ʃ			S	1	1	
*sock	sɑk	sɑk	CVC	1	s	s	k	k	S	2	2	
*zipper	zɪpɚ	dɪpə	CVCV	1	z	d			1	1	2	
hat	hæt	hæt	CVC	1	h	h	t	t	1	2	2	
off	ɑf	ɑf	VC	1			f	f	1	1	1	
# words produced by child/# words possible	15/20		# match 11/15						Total PCC	26	34	

*indicates words acquired between 22–24 months

82

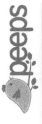
peeps

Word	IPA: Target	IPA: Child	WS Target	WSM	Initial C: Target	Initial C: Child	Final C: Target	Final C: Child	S/I	PCC: Child	PCC: Target	Notes
diaper	daɪpɚ	NR	CVCV	NR	d	NR			NR	NR	~~2~~	
*bib	bɪb	bɪbə	CVC	0	b	b	b	schwa	1	2	2	schwa added
juice	dʒus	du	CVC	0	dʒ	d	s	--	S	2	2	
banana	bənænə	ænænæ	CVCVCV	0	b	n			S	2	3	
cookie	koki	koki	CVCV	1	k	k			S	2	2	
cheese	tʃiz	ti	CVC	1	tʃ	t	z	--	S	0	2	
cup	kʌp	kʌp	CVC	1	k	k	p	p	S	2	2	
drink	dɹɪŋk	dɪŋk	CCVCC	0	dɹ	d	ŋk	ŋk	1	3	4	
bottle	bɑt/dəl	bʌdu	CVCVC	0	b	b	l	vowel	1	2	3	
spoon	spun	bun	CCVC	0	sp	b	n	n	S	1	3	
*train	tɹeɪn	NR	CCVC	NR	tɹ	NR	n	NR	NR	NR	~~3~~	
truck	tɹʌk	tɹʌk	CCVC	1	tɹ	tw	k	k	1	2	3	
*stop	stɑp	NR	CCVC	NR	st	NR	p	NR	NR	NR	~~3~~	
go	goʊ	NR	CV	NR	g	NR			NR	NR	~~1~~	
light	laɪt	lɔaɪ	CVC	1	l	ɔ	t	--	1	0	2	
balloon	bəlun	NR	CVCVC	NR	b	NR	n	NR	NR	NR	~~3~~	
ball	bɑl	bɑ	CVC	0	b	b	l	--	S	1	2	
*rock	ɹɑk	wak	CVC	1	ɹ	ɔ	k	k	1	1	2	
*block	blɑk	bwɑk	CCVC	1	bl	bw	k	k	1	2	3	
*watch	wɑtʃ	wɑts	CVC	1	w	ɔ	tʃ	ts	1	1	2	
# words produced by child / # words possible	15/20		# match	8/15					Total PCC	23	37	

*indicates words acquired between 22–24 months

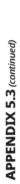

6 Summary of PEEPS Data

Assessment of early phonological skills using PEEPS is intended to provide a descriptive and qualitative analysis that is more appropriate for children ages 18–36 months than a normative and quantitative analysis. The analysis forms yield information on the consonantal inventories, positional patterns of consonants, and word structures produced by the participants. These measures allow clinicians to determine if the inventories are within the expected range for the child's age and expressive vocabulary.

Profiles of early phonological development have been compiled from extensive research studies based on longitudinal and cross-sectional data describing typical phonological acquisition in young children (cf., Dyson, 1988; McIntosh & Dodd, 2008; Scherer et al., 2012; Sosa & Stoel-Gammon, 2012; Stoel-Gammon, 1985, 1987, 1991). The PEEPS summaries below present findings from the seven age groups involved in our study (Williams & Stoel-Gammon, 2016) based on independent and relational analyses.

THE PEEPS DATA SET: SUMMARY AND RESULTS

The PEEPS protocol was administered to children ages 18–36 months, grouped into seven age periods: 18, 21, 24, 27, 30, 33, and 36 months. The data were collected by SLP graduate research assistants in the Department of Audiology and Speech-Language Pathology at East Tennessee State University. According to parental report, all participants were typically developing in terms of speech and language. Data were collected from 10–11 children in each age group and analyzed according to the guidelines presented in the previous chapters.

To be included in the analysis shown here, a participant had to produce a minimum of 10 PEEPS words during the data collection session. At the younger ages, some children did not meet this criterion: two children age 18 months and three children age 21 months produced fewer than 10 words. Thus, the findings presented here are based on data from 67 children in the seven age groups.

Findings: Children Age 18–24 months

Description and analyses of the PEEPS Word List were provided above with an explanation of independent and relational measures. Findings for participants ages 18–24 months are summarized in Table 6.1.

Summary of Findings: Children Age 18–24 Months   As shown in the following table, the data from participants ages 18 and 21 months reveal wide variation in nearly all measures. If we consider the number of words in the samples, we see that the mean number of words produced at 18 months was 22.6 with a range of *12–33* words; at 21 months, the mean was

Table 6.1. Summary of PEEPS findings for children age 18–24 months

Age	18 months (n=8)	21 months (n=7)	24 months (n=10)
Mean # PEEPS Words produced (range)	22.6 (12–33)	27.9 (17–48)	49.5 (29–60)
# Spontaneous Words (range)	12.3 (4–18)	10.9 (2–18)	26.7 (12–42)
Independent Measures			
# Different word-initial Cs (range)	9.6 (5–16)	11.0 (7–17)	13.6 (11–16)
# Different word-final Cs (range)	3.8 (0–8)	6.7 (2–12)	11.6 (8–14)
# Different word-initial clusters (range)	0	0.6 (0–3)	2.5 (0–6)
# Different word-final clusters (range)	0	0.3 (0–1)	1.9 (0–3)
Percentage of Ss producing 2-syllable words	87.5%	85.7%	100%
Percentage of Ss producing 3-syllable words	0	0	20%
Manners of Articulation (# per child; range)			
Mean # different **stop** Cs (range)	4.8 (3–6)	5.1 (3–6)	5.9 (5–6)
Mean # different **fricative** Cs (range)	2.1 (2–4)	3.1 (2–4)	4.1 (3–6)
Mean # different **affricate** Cs (range)	0.9 (0–2)	1.0 (0–2)	0.9 (0–2)
Mean # different **nasal** Cs (range)	1.6 (1–2)	1.9 (1–2)	2.2 (2–3)
Mean # different **liquid** Cs (range)	1.2 (0–2)	1.1 (0–2)	1.6 (1–2)
Mean # different **glide** Cs (range)	1.4 (0–3)	1.4 (0–3)	2.0 (1–3)
Places of Articulation (Percentage of children)	Percentage	Percentage	Percentage
Bilabial	100%	100%	100%
Labiodental	75%	85.7%	100%
Alveolar	100%	100%	100%
Interdental	12.5%	0%	10%
Palatal	87.5%	100%	100%
Velar	87.5%	85.7%	100
Glottal	62.5%	71.4%	90%
Relational Measures			
% Consonants Correct (PCC) (range)	47.5% (35%–68%)	58.3% (32%–83%)	71.3% (55%–87%)
% Word Structure Match (WSM) (range)	41.3% (23%–63%)	48.4% (18%–75%)	68.2% (43%–91%)

27.9 words and the range was *17–48* words. Analyses of individual children show that those participants who produced fewer words have smaller inventories and a reduced variety of word shapes.

General findings for these children are in accordance with typical phonological development, including:

1. Independent Analysis

   • Inventory: A larger inventory of word-initial consonants than word-final consonants

   • Manner: Presence of several stop consonants and few fricatives

   • Place: Presence of the "major" places of articulation: bilabial, alveolar, velar

   • Word Structure: Absence (or very limited occurrence) of consonant clusters in either word-initial or word-final position

2. Relational Analysis: Wide variation in the measures of Percentage of Consonants Correct (PCC) and Word Structure Match (WSM).

At *24 months,* we see a dramatic increase in the number of words produced; the mean number of words produced rises to 49.5, with a range of 29–60. This means that some of the 24-month-old children produced all the words in the PEEPS list. In addition, the phonetic inventory measures increased substantially, with more than 90% of children producing consonants at six of the seven places of articulation. The relational measures also increased over the 6-month period with the PCC rising from 47.5% to 71.3% and the WSM increasing from 41.3% to 68.2%.

Developmental Changes in Profile from 21 Months to 24 Months PEEPS words produced increased significantly from an average of 28 to an average of 49.5 words. The number of words produced spontaneously also increased, from an average of 11 words at 21 months to 26.7 words at 24 months. As shown in Table 6.1, there is still variation in the range of PEEPS words produced (17–48 words at 21 months; 29–60 words at 24 months), as well as in the range of PEEPS words produced spontaneously (2–8 words at 21 months; 12–42 words at 24 months).

General findings for these children align with expected typical phonological development, as noted in the following independent and relational analyses.

1. Independent Analysis

- Consonantal inventories: Substantial increase in number of final consonants

- Manner: Presence of nearly all stop consonants and several fricatives

- Place: Presence of all places of articulation except interdental

- Word Structure: Presence of consonant clusters in both word-initial and word-final position

2. Relational Analysis

- Increase in PCC from mean of 58% to 71%

- Reduced variation across children in PCC measure

- Increase in WSM from mean of 48% to 68%

The developmental changes noted between the younger 18–21 month age group and 24 months represents a clear shift in phonological skills, both quantitative and qualitative. In every measure, 24-month-old children produced more words, had larger phonetic inventories in both word-initial and word-final positions, produced more complex word structures, were more accurate in their productions, and had more stable child:adult correspondences (i.e., less variability). The demarcation between 21 months and 24 months appears to represent a significant shift in phonological development that continues through to 36 months of age.

Findings: Children Age 27–36 months

Findings for participants age 27–36 months are summarized in Table 6.2.

Summary of Findings: Children Age 27–36 Months As shown in the following table, the data for PEEPS words produced ranged from 51 to 56 words. Increases are also evident in the size of phonetic inventories, in the place and manner of articulation, and in the types of syllables structures (production of consonant clusters and of 3-syllable words).

The most notable change in the period from 27 to 36 months is the increase in *accuracy of production.* The measure of PCC rises from a mean of 65% at 27 months to 83% at 36 months, while the mean accuracy of word shapes (WSM) increases from 66% to 87% over the same period.

The increases in accuracy indicate that the participants are using their phonetic skills, as determined by the phonetic inventory measures, in ways that allow them to produce words that conform to the adult targets.

Table 6.2. Summary of PEEPS findings for children age 27–36 months

Age	27 months (n=10)	30 months (n=11)	33 months (n=11)	36 months (n=10)
Mean # PEEPS Words produced (range)	51.1 (33–59)	51.7 (21–60)	54.1 (18–60)	56.1 (47–60)
# Spontaneous Words (range)	25 (6–38)	31.2 (3–45)	34.9 (15–48)	34.9 (22–47)
Independent Measures				
# Different word-initial Cs (range)	14.1 (12–16)	15.0 (10–18)	15.0 (11–17)	15.5 (13–18)
# Different word-final Cs (range)	10.7 (7–16)	13.9 (9–17)	12.1 (4–17)	15.7 (11–20)
# Different word-initial clusters (range)	3.2 (1–6)	3.6 (0–7)	3.9 (0–6)	4.9 (0–6)
# Different word-final clusters (range)	1.6 (0–4)	2.5 (0–4)	2.5 (0–5)	3.2 (0–5)
Percentage of Ss producing 2-sylllable words	100%	100%	100%	100%
Percentage of Ss producing 3-sylllable words	50%	54.50%	54.50%	60%
Manners of Articulation; # per child (range)				
Mean # different **stop** Cs (range)	5.9 (5–7)	5.8 (5–6)	5.6 (5–6)	5.8 (4–6)
Mean # different **fricative** Cs (range)	3.5 (2–5)	3.8 (2–5)	4.2 (2–7)	3.8 (2–5)
Mean # different **affricate** Cs (range)	1.4 (1–2)	1.4 (1–2)	1.3 (0–2)	1.4 (0–2)
Mean # different **nasal** Cs (range)	2.2 (2–3)	2.2 (2–3)	2.5 (2–3)	2.5 (2–3)
Mean # different **liquid** Cs (range)	1.7 (1–3)	1.6 (1–2)	1.4 (1–2)	1.4 (0–2)
Mean # different **glide** Cs (range)	2.1 (1–3)	2.1 (1–3)	1.5 (0–2)	1.6 (1–2)
Places of articulation (% children)	Percentage	Percentage	Percentage	Percentage
Bilabial	100%	100%	100%	100%
Labiodental	100%	100%	100%	100%
Alveolar	100%	100%	100%	100%
Interdental	10%	45.4%	36.3%	40%
Palatal	100%	100%	100%	90%
Velar	100%	90.9%	90.9%	90%
Glottal	100%	100%	100%	100%
Relational Measures				
% Consonants Correct (PCC) (range)	65.1% (43%–88%)	83.7% (70%–93%)	76.7% (48%–94%)	83.3% (64%–95%)
% Word Structure Match (WSM) (range)	65.9% (26%–88%)	83.4% (72%–92%)	75.6% (28%–97%)	87.6% (70%–98%)

Aspects of the findings from the PEEPS data set are in accordance with expected development, as summarized below.

Independent Analysis

- Inventory:
    - Word-initial inventory large at all ages
    - Word-final inventory increases with age
    - Number of word-initial and word-final clusters increases with age
- Manner: Nearly all manner classes present at all ages, except affricates and liquids
- Place: All place classes, except interdental, are present

- Word Structure:
  - All children produce 2-syllable words
  - More than half the children produce 3-syllable words

Relational Analysis

- PCC increases from mean of 65% at 27 months to 83% at 36 months
- WSM increases from mean of 66% at 27 months to 88% at 36 months
- Variability of WSM across children decreases

SUMMARY

PEEPS data were presented on typically developing children between 18 months and 36 months of age divided into seven age groups: 18, 21, 24, 27, 30, 33, and 36 months. Several measures were summarized across the age groups, including phonetic inventory (number of consonants by word position; place, voice, manner of consonants produced); word/syllable structure; accuracy; and word shape matches. A demarcation of development was noted between younger children 18–21 months and older children 24 months and older across all measures, including number of words produced, less variability, larger phonetic inventories, more complex word structures, and more accurate productions.

Age of Acquisition of PEEPS Words

PEEPS Target Word	% acquired: 18 months	% acquired: 21 months	% acquired: 24 months
baby	75	85	91
ball	90	94	96
balloon	60	71	87
banana	66	77	87
belly button	<50	57	75
bib	<50	<50	57
bird	62	75	87
blanket	<50	58	79
block	<50	<50	67
bottle	<50	61	73
bug	<50	50	73
cheese	57	67	87
chicken	<50	<50	64
comb	<50	<50	50
cookie	57	70	87
cow	<50	54	79
cup	<50	64	81
diaper	<50	69	81
dog	78	85	93
doll	<50	<50	63
drink	<50	51	77
duck	61	67	88
ear	59	75	87
elephant	<50	<50	67

PEEPS Target Word	% acquired: 18 months	% acquired: 21 months	% acquired: 24 months
finger	<50	52	73
foot	<50	<50	76
go	<50	67	82
hair	<50	67	82
hand	<50	57	74
hat	54	69	74
juice	58	76	87
kitty	60	69	79
light	<50	55	77
lion	<50	<50	64
monkey	<50	<50	75
moo	71	76	90
mouse	<50	<50	62
mouth	<50	57	79
nose	65	76	91
off	<50	<50	51
peek-a-boo	<50	58	77
pig	<50	50	77
puppy	<50	54	73
quack	58	62	83
rock	<50	<50	67
sheep	<50	<50	60
shoe	76	81	94
soap	<50	<50	68
sock	<50	<50	72
spoon	<50	62	78
stop	<50	<50	66
toe	<50	54	72
tongue	<50	<50	59
train	<50	<50	79
truck	51	65	85
tummy	<50	<50	73

PEEPS Target Word	% acquired: 18 months	% acquired: 21 months	% acquired: 24 months
watch	<50	<50	52
woof	72	75	88
zipper	<50	<50	51

Key: AoA, Age of Acquisition.

AoA 18 mos (n=19): baby, ball, balloon, banana, bird, cheese, cookie, dog, duck, ear, hat, juice, kitty, moo, nose, quack, shoe, truck, woof

AoA 21 mos (n=20): bed, bellybutton, blanket, bottle, bug, cow, cup, diaper, drink, finger, go, hair, hand, light, mouth, peek-a-boo, pig, puppy, spoon, toe

AoA 24 mos (n=21): bib, block, chicken, comb, doll, elephant, foot, lion, monkey, mouse, off, rock, sheep, soap, sock, stop, tongue, train, tummy, watch, zipper

B Summaries of PEEPS Data for Children Ages 18–36 Months: Individual Data

Key:

#wds, number of words produced; **#sp wds, number of spontaneous words; % PCC,** percentage of consonants correct; **% WSM,** percentage of word structure matches; **#WI Cons,** number of word-initial consonants; **#WF Cons,** number of word-final consonants; **2Sy,** child produced 2-syllable words; **3Sy,** child produced 3-syllable words

18M (8)	#wds	#sp wds	% PCC	% WSM	#WI Cons	#WF Cons		2Sy	3Sy
	16	11	44	63	8	3		Y	N
	13	13	38	23	5	0		Y	N
	27	17	36	30	10	5		Y	N
	33	15	49	39	16	5		Y	N
	29	18	55	45	10	4		N	N
	24	12	55	42	11	3		Y	N
	12	4	35	25	6	2		Y	N
	27	8	68	63	11	8		Y	N
MEANS	22.6	12.3	47.5	41.3	9.6	3.8		Total	Total
Range	12 < 33	4 < 18	35 < 68	23 < 63	5 < 16	0 < 8		7	0

21M (7)	#wds	#sp wds	% PCC	% WSM	#WI Cons	#WF Cons	2Sy	3Sy
	29	7	55	59	7	8	Y	N
	17	16	32	18	7	2	Y	N
	32	16	59	34	14	5	N	N
	20	5	62	60	8	7	Y	N
	20	2	63	45	12	4	Y	N
	48	18	83	75	17	12	Y	N
	29	12	54	48	12	9	Y	N
MEANS	27.9	10.9	58.3	48.4	11.0	6.7	Total	Total
Range	17 < 48	2 < 18	32 < 83	18 < 75	7 < 17	2 < 12	6	0

24M (10)	#wds	#sp wds	% PCC	% WSM	#WI Cons	#WF Cons	2Sy	3Sy
	36	12	65	64	13	10	Y	N
	55	26	60	56	11	13	Y	N
	46	19	56	43	13	8	N	N
	60	42	81	80	16	13	Y	Y
	58	29	87	91	15	14	Y	Y
	55	32	80	76	14	12	Y	N
	51	31	74	76	13	13	Y	N
	49	27	80	80	14	12	Y	N
	29	15	55	48	11	8	Y	N
	56	34	75	68	16	13	Y	N
MEANS	49.5	26.7	71.3	68.2	13.6	11.6	Total	Total
Range	29 < 60	12 < 42	55 < 87	43 < 91	11 < 16	8 < 14	10	2

27M (10)	#wds	#sp wds	% PCC	% WSM	#WI Cons	#WF Cons	2Sy	3Sy
	56	29	66	68	13	11	Y	Y
	59	33	78	88	14	16	Y	Y
	33	18	53	64	13	7	N	N
	56	31	44	45	12	9	Y	N
	54	38	72	76	15	13	Y	N
	59	27	81	83	16	11	Y	Y
	40	22	53	60	14	10	Y	Y
	47	6	43	26	13	7	Y	N
	50	24	88	66	16	11	Y	N
	57	22	73	83	15	12	Y	Y
MEANS	51.1	25	65.1	65.9	14.1	10.7	Total	Total
Range	40 < 59	6 < 38	43 < 88	26 < 88	12 < 16	7 < 16	10	5

30M (11)	#wds	@sp wds	% PCC	% WSM	#WI Cons	#WF Cons	2Sy	3Sy
	58	40	90	84	17	16	Y	N
	58	38	83	72	16	13	Y	Y
	59	24	90	90	18	17	Y	Y
	60	38	94	92	16	15	Y	Y
	59	45	82	92	14	12	Y	Y
	60	41	93	92	17	17	Y	N
	60	37	80	82	13	16	Y	N
	55	34	72	75	16	14	Y	Y
	21	3	82	76	10	9	Y	N
	29	14	85	76	13	11	Y	Y
	50	29	70	86	15	13	Y	N
MEANS	51.7	31.2	83.7	83.4	15.0	13.9	Total	Total
Range	29 < 60	3 < 45	70 < 94	72 < 92	10 < 18	9 < 17	11	6

30M (11)	#wds	#sp wds	% PCC	% WSM	#WI Cons	#WF Cons	2Sy	3Sy
	58	40	90	84	17	16	Y	N
	58	38	83	72	16	13	Y	Y
	59	24	90	90	18	17	Y	Y
	60	38	94	92	16	15	Y	Y
	59	45	82	92	14	12	Y	Y
	60	41	93	92	17	17	Y	N
	60	37	80	82	13	16	Y	N
	55	34	72	75	16	14	Y	Y
	21	3	82	76	10	9	Y	N
	29	14	85	76	13	11	Y	Y
	50	29	70	86	15	13	Y	N
MEANS	51.7	31.2	83.7	83.4	15.0	13.9	Total	Total
Range	29 < 60	3 < 45	70 < 94	72 < 92	10 < 18	9 < 17	11	6

36M (10)	#wds	#sp wds	% PCC	% WSM	#WI Cons	#WF Cons	2Sy	3Sy
	60	42	58	70	13	14	Y	Y
	57	35	84	93	14	19	Y	N
	57	38	95	93	18	15	Y	Y
	60	36	64	78	15	17	Y	Y
	47	31	91	87	15	14	Y	Y
	59	32	72	83	16	19	Y	Y
	52	40	94	98	16	16	Y	Y
	60	37	94	87	17	16	T	N
	54	47	94	98	15	15	Y	N
	55	22	87	89	16	11	Y	Y
MEANS	56.1	36	83.3	87.6	15.5	15.6	Total	Total
Range	47 < 60	22 < 47	64 < 95	70 < 98	13 < 18	11 < 19	10	6

Children's Speech Development

Sharynne McLeod, Ph.D.
Charles Sturt University, Australia

This compilation of data on typical speech development for English-speaking children is designed to be used by speech-language pathologists. It is organized according to children's ages to reflect a typical developmental sequence. However, it should be noted that rates of development vary among typically developing children. Where possible, data from more than one study is presented under each heading at each age to allow for comparison and to encourage consideration of diversity and individuality.

Authors	Year	Country	No. of children	Age of children	Sample type	Data collection method
Anthony, Bogle, Ingram, & McIsaac	1971	UK	510	3;0–6;0	SW	Cross-sectional
Arlt & Goodban	1976	USA	240	3;0–5;5	Single word (SW)	Cross-sectional
Chirlian & Sharpley	1982	Australia	1357	2;6–9;0	Single word (SW)	Cross-sectional
Dodd	1995	UK & Australia	5	1;8–3;0	Connected speech	Longitudinal
Dodd, Holm, Hua, & Crosbie	2003	UK	684	3;0–6;11	SW	Cross-sectional
Donegan	2002	UK & USA	–	–	–	Compilation
Dyson	1988	USA	20	2;0–3;3	CS	Cross-sectional & longitudinal
Flipsen	2006a, b	USA	320	3;1–8;10	CS	Cross-sectional
Grunwell	1987	UK	–	–	–	Compilation
Haelsig & Madison	1986	USA	50	2;10–5;2	SW	Cross-sectional
James	2001	Australia	354	3;0–7;11	SW	Cross-sectional

(continued)

Printed by permission of Sharynne McLeod, as adapted by Sharynne McLeod from McLeod, S., & Bleile, K. (2003, November). *Neurological and developmental foundations of speech acquisition. A summary: brain development and the environment* [Paper presentation]. American Speech-Language-Hearing Association Convention, Chicago, IL, United States.

Authors	Year	Country	No. of children	Age of children	Sample type	Data collection method
James, van Doorn, & McLeod	2001	Australia	354	3;0–7;11	SW	Cross-sectional
James, van Doorn, & McLeod	2002	Australia	354	3;0–7;11	SW	Cross-sectional
Kehoe	1997	USA	18	1;10–2;10	SW	Cross-sectional
Kehoe	2001	USA	–	1;6–2;10	–	Compilation
Kilminster & Laird	1978	Australia	1756	3;0–9;0	SW	Cross-sectional
Lowe, Knutson & Monson	1985	USA	1048	2;7–4;6	SW	Cross-sectional
McGlaughlin & Grayson	2003	UK	297	0;1–1;0	Crying	Cross-sectional
McLeod, van Doorn, & Reed	2001a	Australia	–	–	–	Compilation
McLeod, van Doorn, & Reed	2001b	Australia	16	2;0–3;4	CS	Longitudinal
McLeod, van Doorn, & Reed	2002	Australia	16	2;0–3;4	CS	Longitudinal
Oller, Eilers, Neal, & Schwartz	1999	USA	3400	0;10–1;0	CS; Parent report	Cross-sectional & longitudinal
Otomo & Stoel-Gammon	1992	USA	6	1;10–2;6	SW	Longitudinal
Paynter & Petty	1974	USA	90	2;0–2;6	SW	Cross-sectional
Pollock	2002	USA (Memphis)	162	1;6–6;10	SW & CS	Cross-sectional
Pollock & Berni	2003	USA (Memphis)	165	1;6–6;10	SW & CS	Cross-sectional
Porter & Hodson	2001	USA	520	2;6–8;0	SW	Cross-sectional
Prather, Hedrick, & Kern	1975	USA	147	2;0–4;0	SW	Cross-sectional
Preisser, Hodson, & Paden	1988	USA	60	1;6–2;5	SW	Cross-sectional
Robb & Bleile	1994	USA	7	0;8–2;1	CS	Longitudinal
Robb & Gillon	2007	New Zealand & USA	20	3;1–3;5 (NZ) 2;11–3;5 (US)	CS	Cross-sectional
Robbins & Klee	1987	USA	90	2;6–6;11	SW	Cross-sectional
Roberts, Burchinal, & Footoo	1990	USA	145	2;6–8;0	SW	Cross-sectional & longitudinal
Roulstone, Loader, Northstone, Beveridge, & ALSPAC team	2002	UK	1127	2;1	SW; Parent report	Single age group
Selby, Robb, & Gilbert	2000	USA	4	1;3–3;0	CS	Longitudinal

Authors	Year	Country	No. of children	Age of children	Sample type	Data collection method
Shriberg	1993	USA	-	-	-	Compilation
Smit	1993b	USA	997	3;0–9;0	SW	Cross-sectional
Smit	1993a	USA	997	3;0–9;0	SW	Cross-sectional
Smit, Hand, Frelinger, Bernthal, & Bird	1990	USA	997	3;0–9;0	SW	Cross-sectional
Stoel-Gammon	1985	USA	34	1;3–2;0	CS	Longitudinal
Stoel-Gammon	1987	USA	33	2;0	CS	Cross-sectional
Stokes	2005	USA	40	2;1	CS	Single age group
Watson & Scukanec	1997a, b	USA	12	2;0–3;0	CS	Longitudinal

GLOSSARY: Acquired sounds = The age at which a certain percentage (often 75%) of children have acquired a phoneme in initial, medial, and final position in single words. **Phonetic inventory** = Repertoire of sounds a child can produce, regardless of the adult target. **Syllable shape** = Structure of a syllable within a word. **C** = consonant. **V** = vowel.

0;0 – 1;0 year

"The interaction between infants and their caregivers lays so many foundations for later learning" (McLaughlin, 1998, p. 192).

PERCEPTION

"By at least 2 days of age, the neonate has an ability to discriminate language specific acoustic distinctions ... The 12 month old human has developed the capacity to categorise only those phonemes which are in its native language."

(Ruben, 1997, p. 203)

CRYING

Mean amount of crying/ 24 hours

1–3 months = 90 mins, mostly in the evening
4–6 months = 64.7 mins, mostly afternoon
7–9 months = 60.5 mins, afternoon/evening
10–12 months = 86.4 mins, mostly evening
Other studies show decrease at 10+ months

(McGlaughlin & Grayson, 2003)

VOCALIZATION

0–6 weeks = reflexive vocalisations: cry, fuss
6–16 weeks = coo and laughter: vowel-like
16–30 weeks = syllable-like vocalizations

(Stark, Bernstein, & Demorest, 1983)

0–0;2 = phonation, quasivowels & glottals
0;2–0;3 = primitive articulation stage: gooing
0;4–0;5 = expansion stage: full vowels, raspberries, marginal babbling

(Oller, Eilers, Neal, & Schwartz, 1999)

BABBLING

"Late onset of canonical babbling may be a predictor of disorders ... [i.e.] smaller production vocabularies at 18, 24 & 36 months"

(Oller, Eilers, Neal, & Schwartz, 1999, p. 223).

31–50 weeks = reduplicated babbling: series of consonant and vowel-like elements

(Mitchell, 1997; Stark, 1979)

0;6+ = canonical stage: well-formed canonical syllables, reduplicated sequences (e.g., [bababa])

(Oller et al., 1999)

"The sounds babbled most frequently are produced more accurately by English-learning 2-year-olds, and appear more often in the languages of the world, than other sounds"

(Locke, 2002, p. 249).

PHONETIC INVENTORY

Consonants

Nasal, plosive, fricative, approximant, labial, lingual

(Grunwell, 1981)

1;0 = Mean 4.4 consonants; median 4; range 0–16

(Ttofari-Eecen et al., 2007)

1;0 = /m, d, b, n/ most frequently reported consonants in inventory

(Ttofari-Eecen et al., 2007)

0;8 = 5 consonants in initial position (typically /d, t, k, m, h/); 3 consonants in final position (typically /t, m, h/)
0;9 = 5 consonants in initial position (typically /d, m, n,

h, w/); 2 consonants in final position (typically /m, h/)
0;10 = 6 consonants in initial position (typically /b, d, t, m, n, h/); 4 consonants in final position (typically /t, m, h, s/)
0;11 = 4 consonants in initial position (typically /d, m, n, h/); 2 consonants in final position (typically /m, h/)
1;0 = 5 consonants in initial position (typically / b, d, g, m, h/); 2 consonants in final position (typically /m, h/)

(Robb & Bleile, 1994)

Vowels

"Low, non-rounded vowels are favoured in the first year. Front-back vowel differences appear later than height differences"

(Donegan, 2002).

PHONOLOGICAL PROCESSES

Present

All phonological processes
(Grunwell, 1987)

SYLLABLE STRUCTURE

Primarily mono-syllabic utterances

(Bauman-Waengler, 2000, p. 99)

PROSODY

0;10–1;0 = Begin with falling contour only. Flat or level contour, usually accompanied by variations such as falsettos or variations in duration of loudness

(Marcos, 1987 adapted by Bauman-Waengler, 2000)

1;0 - 2;0 years

"...from 18 to 24 months ... the largest growth within the phonological system takes place ... also ... the child's expressive vocabulary has at least tripled" (Bauman-Waengler, 2000, p. 107).

ORAL MECHANISM

Deciduous teeth continue to emerge

INTELLIGIBILITY

2;0 = 26%–50% intelligible
(Weiss, 1982)

ACQUIRED SOUNDS

Consonants (females)

2;0 = /m, n, h, g/
(Chirlian & Sharpley, 1982)

Consonants (males)

2;0 = /m, n/
(Chirlian & Sharpley, 1982)

Consonants (all children)

2;0 = /h, w/
(Paynter & Petty, 1974)

2;0 = /m, n, ŋ, h, p/
(Prather, Hedrick, & Kern, 1975)

Consonant clusters

?

Vowels

?

PERCENT CORRECT

Consonants

2;0 = 69.2 (range 53–91)
(Watson & Scukanec, 1997b)

Consonant clusters

?

Vowels (USA - nonrhotic)

1;6–1;11 = 82% (range = 69–96)
(Pollock & Berni, 2003)

COMMON MISMATCHES

Consonants

?

Consonant clusters

?

PHONOLOGICAL PROCESSES

Present

Final consonant deletion, cluster reduction, fronting of velars, stopping, gliding, context sensitive voicing
(Grunwell, 1987)

Declining

Reduplication, consonant harmony
(Grunwell, 1987)

PHONETIC INVENTORY

"First words show individual variation in consonants used; phonetic variability in pronunciations"
(Grunwell, 1987)

Consonants

/m, p, b, w, n, t, d/
(Grunwell, 1987)

1;0 = 5 consonants in initial position (typically /b, d, g, m, h/); 2 consonants in final position (typically /m, h/)

1;6 = 6 consonants in initial position (typically /b, d, m, n, h, w/); 3 consonants in final position (typically /t, h, s/)

2;0 = 10 consonants in initial position (typically /b, d, p, t, k, m, n, h, s, w/); 4 consonants in final position (typically /t, k, n, s/)
(Robb & Bleile, 1994)

1;0 – Mean = 4.4 consonants; median = 4; range 0–16

1;0 – /m, d, b, n/ most frequently reported consonants in inventory
(Ttofari-Eecen et al., 2007)

Vowels (USA)

1;3 = /ɪ, ʊ, ʌ, ɑ/
1;6 = /i, u, ʊ, ʌ, ɔ, ɑ, æ/
1;9 = /i, ɪ, u, ɛ, o, ʌ, ɔ, ɑ/
2;0 = /i, ɪ, u, ɛ, e, o, ɔ, ɑ, æ/
(Selby, Robb, & Gilbert, 2000)

SYLLABLE STRUCTURE

?

PROSODY

Young children acquire skills that control intonation earlier than final syllable timing skills
(Snow, 1994).

1;1–1;3 = Rising contour. High falling contour that begins with a high pitch and drops to a lower one prior to 1;6 = high rising and high rising-falling contour around 1;6 = falling-rising contour. Rising-falling contour
(Marcos, 1987; adapted by Bauman-Waengler, 2000)

METALINGUISTIC SKILLS

1;6–2;0 = monitor own utterances: repair spontaneously, adjust speech to different listeners, practice sounds, words, sentences
(Clark, adapted by Owens, 1996, p. 386)

2;0 – 3;0 years

"Unlike toddlers, preschoolers develop more freedom of movement and therefore, soon become trailblazers in every sense of the word" (McLaughlin, 1998, p. 271).

"A client 3 years of age or older who is unintelligible is a candidate for treatment" (Bernthal & Bankson, 1998, p. 272).

ORAL MECHANISM

During first 3 years of life:

Oral space enlarges. Growth of lower jaw + other bony structures. Increased muscle tone and "skilled" tongue movement.
Lowering & more sophisticated movement of larynx. Separation of epiglottis & soft palate.

DDK (2;6 – 2;11)

/pʌ/ = 3.7 per second; /tʌ/ = 3.7 per second
/kʌ/ = 3.65 per second; patti-cake = 1.26/sec
(Robbins & Klee, 1987)

Maximum phonation time

2;6–2;11 = 5.55/sec
(Robbins & Klee, 1987)

INTELLIGIBILITY

2;1 = "… children were mostly intelligible to their parents with 12.7% parents finding their child difficult to understand and only 2.1% of parents reporting that they could rarely understand their child"
(Roulstone et al., 2002, p. 264)

3;0 = 95.68% (88.89–100.00) % of words that could be reliably understood by the transcriber
(Flipsen, 2006b)

2;0 = 26%–50% intelligible
2;6 = 51%–70% intelligible
3;0 = 71%–80% intelligible
(Weiss, 1982)

3;0 = 73% (50%–80%) intelligible judged by three unfamiliar listeners. The children who used more complex sentences were more difficult to understand
(Vihman, 1988)

ACQUIRED SOUNDS

Consonants (females)

≤3;0 = /m, n, h, w, p, b, t, d, k, g, f/
3;0 = + /s/
(Smit et al., 1990)

2;0 = /m, n, h, g/
2;6 = + /p, ŋ, w, t, d, k/
3;0 = + /j, f/
(Chirlian & Sharpley, 1982)

3;0 = /h, ŋ, p, m, w, b, n, d, t, k, ʒ, f/
(Kilminster & Laird, 1978)

Consonants (males)

≤3;0 & 3;0 = /m, n, h, w, p, b, t, d, k, g/
(Smit et al., 1990)

2;0 = /m, n/
2;6 = + /ŋ, d/
3;0 = +/p, b, h, w, k, g/
(Chirlian & Sharpley, 1982)

3;0 = /h, ŋ, p, m, w, b, n, d, j, g, ʒ/
(Kilminster & Laird, 1978)

Consonants (all children)

2;0 = /h, w/
2;6 = +/p, b, t, m/
(Paynter & Petty, 1974)

2;0 = /m, n, ŋ, h, p/
2;4 = +/j, d, k, f/
2;8 = +/w, b, t/
3;0 = +/g, s/
(Prather, Hedrick, & Kern, 1975)

3;0 = /p, b, t, d, k, g, m, n, ŋ, h, f, w/
(Arlt & Goodban, 1976)

3;0 = /p, b, t, d, k, g, m, n, ŋ, f, v, s, z, h, w, l, j/
(Dodd et al., 2003)

Consonant clusters

"Two-year-old children can produce consonant clusters, but these may not be of the same form as the ambient language"
(McLeod, van Doorn & Reed, 2001a).

Vowels

"The literature on vowel development suggests that vowels are acquired early, both in production and perception. There is considerable variability in their production, but most studies suggest that vowel production is reasonably accurate by age 3, although some studies call this into question."
(Donegan, 2002, p. 2)

1;10–2;6 = /i, ɑ/ mastered early, /ɛ, æ/ next, /ɪ, ɛ/ least accurate
(Otomo & Stoel-Gammon, 1992)

PERCENT CORRECT

Consonants

PCC = 70%
(Stoel-Gammon, 1987)

2;0 = 69.2% (range 53–91)
2;3 = 69.9% (range 51–91)

2;6 = 75.1% (range 61–94)
2;9 = 82.1% (range 63–96)
3;0 = 86.2% (range 73–99)
(Watson & Scukanec, 1997b)

3;0–3;11 = 82.11%
(Dodd et al., 2003)

Consonant clusters

2;0–3;4 = 29.5% (mean);
0.0–79.1% (range) in
conversational speech
(McLeod, van Doorn, &
Reed, 2001b)

Vowels (UK)

3;0–3;11 = 97.39%
(Dodd et al., 2003)

Vowels (USA - nonrhotic)

2;0–2;5 = 92.4% (range = 78–100)
2;6–2;11 = 93.9% (range = 78–100)
(Pollock, 2002;
Pollock & Berni, 2003)

Vowels (USA - rhotic)

2;0–2;5 = 37.5% (range = 0–87)
2;6–2;11 = 62.5% (range = 0–100)
(Pollock, 2002)

PERCENT ERROR

Consonants

2;7 = mean error rate for velars
= 31%
2;7 = mean error rate for
fricatives = 38%
2;7 = mean error rate for
liquids = 57%
(Roulstone et al.,
2002)

Consonant clusters

2;7 = mean error rate 72%
(Roulstone et al.,
2002)

COMMON MISMATCHES

Consonants (>15%)

ŋ→ n; j→ Ø; l→ w; r→ w; v→b;
θ→f; ð→ d; s→ dentalised; z→d;
ʃ→ s; tʃ→ t/d; ʒ→d
(Smit, 1993a)

Consonant clusters (>15%)

pr→p, pw; br→b, bw; tr→t, tw;
dr→d, dw; kr→k, kw; gr→g,
gw; fr→f, fw; θr→f, θw; sw→w;
sm→m; sn→n; sp→p, b; st→t, d;
sk→k, skw→k, t, kw, gw; spl→p,
b, pl, pw; spr→p, pw, pr, sp;
str→t, d, st, tw, sw; skr→k, w,
kw, gw, fw
(Smit, 1993b)

PHONOLOGICAL PROCESSES

Present

Cluster reduction, fronting of
velars, fronting /ʃ/, stopping /v,
θ, ð tʃ, dʒ/, gliding, context sensitive voicing
(Grunwell, 1987)

Most prevalent = cluster
reduction & liquid deviations
(gliding)
(Preisser et al., 1988)

2;0 = final consonant deletion,
liquid simplification, later
stopping, cluster reduction,
vowelisation
3;0 = later stopping, cluster
simplification
(Watson & Scukanec,
1997b)

2;7–3;0 = 23% fronting
(Lowe, Knutson & Monson,
1985)

Declining

Final consonant deletion
(Grunwell, 1987)
Affrication, depalatisation,
gliding, meathesis, prevocalic
voicing, vowel changes
(James, 2001)

PHONETIC INVENTORY

Consonants (word-initial)

9–10 consonants
(Stoel-Gammon, 1987)
2;0 = /p, b, t, d, k, m, n, s, f, h,
w, j/

2;3 = /p, b, t, d, k, g, m, n, s, f, h,
w, j, l/
2;6 = /p, b, t, d, k, g, m, n, s, f, h,
tʃ, w, j, l/
2;9 = /p, b, t, d, k, g, m, n, s, f, h,
tʃ, w, j, l/
3;0 = /p, b, t, d, k, g, m, n, s, f, h,
tʃ, ð, w, j, l/
(Watson & Scukanec,
1997b)

/m, p, b, w, n, t, d, (ŋ), (k), (g), h/
(Grunwell, 1987)

2;0, 2;5, 2;9 = /p, b, t, d, k, g, f, s,
h, m, n, w, j, l/
(Dyson, 1988)

Consonants (word-final)

5–6 final consonants
(Stoel-Gammon, 1987)

2;0 = /p, t, k, m, n, s, z/
2;3 = /p, t, d, m, n, s, z/
2;6, 2;9, 3;0 = /p, t, d, k, m, n, s,
z, l, r/
(Watson & Scukanec,
1997b)

2;0 = /p, t, d, k, tʃ, ʔ, f, s, ʃ, m, n/
2;5 = /p, t, d, k, tʃ, ʔ, f, s, ʃ, m, n,
ŋ, ɚ/
2;9 = /p, t, k, ʔ, f, s, ʃ, m, n, ɚ/
(Dyson, 1988)

Consonant clusters

"A few clusters"
(Stoel-Gammon, 1987)

2;6 = /pw, bw, -nd, -ts/
2;9 = /pw, bw, bl, -nd, -ts, -nt, -nz/
3;0 = /st, sp, pl, -nd, -ts, -nt, -nz,
-st, -mk/
(Watson & Scukanec,
1997b)

2;0 = /fw, -ts (-ŋk)/
2;5 = /(fw), (bw), -ts, (-ps), (ntʃ),
(ŋk)/
2;9 = /(fw), (kw), (-ps), (-ts), (-nts),
(-ŋk)/
(Dyson, 1988)

2;0 = predominantly word-
initial consonant clusters containing /w/ (e.g., [bw, kw])

3;0 = range of word-initial clusters predominantly containing /l/, /w/ or /s/.

Common word-final clusters contained nasals (e.g., [-nd, -nt, -ŋk]).

(McLeod, van Doorn, & Reed, 2001b)

Vowels

2;0 = /i, ɪ, u, ɛ, e, o, ɔ, ɑ, æ/
3;0 = /i, ɪ, u, ʊ, ɛ, e, o, ʌ, ɔ, ɜ, ɑ, æ/
(Selby, Robb, & Gilbert, 2000)

SYLLABLE STRUCTURE

Syllable shapes

CV, CVC, CVCV, CVCVC
(Stoel-Gammon, 1987)
CV, VC, CVC, 2-syllable
(Shriberg, 1993)
Monosyllabic words - V, CV, VC, CVC, CCVC, CVCC, CCVCC, CCVCCC, CCCCVC
Polysyllabic words - V, CV, VC, CVC, CCVC
(Dodd, 1995; Watson & Skucanec, 1997)

PROSODY

"Significantly greater number of stress errors in SWS words (S = strong; W = weak). Tendency for greater number of stress errors in SWSW words. Stress errors were more frequent in imitated than spontaneous productions."

(Kehoe, 1997)

"An analysis of children's truncation error syllable deletion patterns revealed the following robust findings:

a. Stressed and word-final unstressed syllables are preserved more frequently than nonfinal unstressed syllables,
b. word-internal unstressed syllables with obstruent onsets are preserved more frequently than word-internal syllables with sonorant onsets,
c. unstressed syllables with non-reduced vowels are preserved more frequently than unstressed syllables with reduced vowels,
d. right-sided stressed syllables are preserved more frequently than left-sided stressed syllables.

An analysis of children's stress patterns revealed that children made greater numbers of stress errors in target words with irregular stress."

(Kehoe, 2001, p. 284)

METALINGUISTIC SKILLS

1;6–2;0 = monitor own utterances: repair spontaneously, adjust speech to different listeners, practice sounds, words, sentences

(Clark, adapted by Owens, 1996, p. 386)

Appendix C References

Bauman-Waengler, J. (2000). *Articulation and phonological impairments: A clinical focus.* Allyn & Bacon.

Bernthal, J. E., & Bankson, N. W. (1998). *Articulation and phonological disorders* (4th ed.). Allyn & Bacon.

Chirlian, N. S., & Sharpley, C. F. (1982). Children's articulation development: Some regional differences. *Australian Journal of Human Communication Disorders, 10,* 23–30.

Dodd, B. (1995). Children's acquisition of phonology. In B. Dodd (Ed.), *Differential diagnosis and treatment of speech disordered children* (pp. 21–48). Whurr.

Dodd, B., & Gillon, G. (2001). Exploring the relationship between phonological awareness, speech impairment, and literacy. *Advances in Speech-Language Pathology, 3,* 139–147.

Donegan, P. (2002). Normal vowel development. In M. J. Ball & F. E. Gibbon (Eds.), *Vowel disorders* (pp. 1–35). Butterworth-Heinemann.

Dyson, A. T. (1988). Phonetic inventories of 2- and 3-year-old children. *Journal of Speech and Hearing Disorders, 53,* 89–93.

Gordon-Brannan, M. (1994). Assessing intelligibility: Children's expressive phonologies. *Topics in Language Disorders, 14,* 17–25.

Grunwell, P. (1981). The development of phonology: A descriptive profile. *First Language, 3,* 161–191.

Grunwell, P. (1987). *Clinical phonology* (2nd ed.). Croom Helm.

Haelsig, P. C., & Madison, C. L. (1986). A study of phonological processes exhibited by 3-, 4-, and 5-year-old children. *Language, Speech, and Hearing Services in Schools, 17,* 107–114.

James, D. G. H. (2001). The use of phonological processes in Australian children aged 2 to 7:11 years. *Advances in Speech-Language Pathology, 3,* 109–128.

James, D., van Doorn, J., & McLeod, S. (2001). Vowel production in mono-, di- and poly-syllabic words in children 3;0 to 7;11 years. In L. Wilson & S. Hewat (Eds.), *Proceedings of the Speech Pathology Australia Conference* (pp. 127–136). Speech Pathology Australia.

James, D., van Doorn, J., & McLeod, S. (2002). Segment production in mono-, di- and polysyllabic words in children aged 3–7 years. In F. Windsor, L. Kelly, & N. Hewlett (Eds.), *Themes in Clinical Phonetics and Linguistics* (pp. 287– 298). Lawrence Erlbaum.

Kehoe, M. (1997). Stress error patterns in English-speaking children's word productions. *Clinical Linguistics and Phonetics, 11,* 389–409.

Kehoe, M. M. (2001). Prosodic patterns in children's multisyllabic word productions. *Language, Speech, and Hearing Services in Schools, 32,* 284–294.

Kilminster, M. G. E., & Laird, E. M. (1978). Articulation development in children aged three to nine years. *Australian Journal of Human Communication Disorders, 6,* 23–30.

Locke, J. L. (2002). Vocal development in the human infant: Functions and phonetics. In F. Windsor, M. L. Kelly, & N. Hewlett (Eds.), *Investigations in clinical phonetics and linguistics* (pp. 243–256). Lawrence Erlbaum.

Lowe, R. J., Knutson, P. J., & Monson, M. A. (1985). Incidence of fronting in preschool children. *Language, Speech, and Hearing Services in Schools, 16,* 119–123.

McGlaughlin, A., & Grayson, A. (2003). A cross sectional and prospective study of crying in the first year of life. In S. P. Sohov (Ed.), *Advances in Psychology Research* (Vol. 22, pp. 37–58). Nova Science.

McLaughlin, S. (1998). *Introduction to language development.* Singular.

McLeod, S. (2002). Part I: The plethora of available data on children's speech development. *ACQuiring Knowledge in Speech, Language and Hearing, 4,* 141–147.

McLeod, S. (2003). General trends and individual differences: Perspectives on normal speech development. In S. P. Sohov (Ed.), *Advances in Psychology Research* (Vol. 22, pp. 189–202). New York: Nova Science.

McLeod, S., van Doorn, J., & Reed, V. A. (2001a). Normal acquisition of consonant clusters. *American Journal of Speech-Language Pathology, 10,* 99–110.

McLeod, S., van Doorn, J., & Reed, V. A. (2001b). Consonant cluster development in two-year-olds: General trends and individual difference. *Journal of Speech, Language, Hearing Research, 44,* 1144–1171.

McLeod, S., van Doorn, J., & Reed, V. A. (2002). Typological description of the normal acquisition of consonant clusters. In F. Windsor, L. Kelly, & N. Hewlett (Eds.), *Themes in clinical phonetics and linguistics* (pp. 185–200). Lawrence Erlbaum.

Mitchell, P. R. (1997). Prelinguistic vocal development: A clinical primer. *Contemporary Issues in Communication Science and Disorders, 24,* 87–92.

Oller, D. K., Eilers, R. E., Neal, A. R., & Schwartz, H. K. (1999). Precursors to speech in infancy: The prediction of speech and language disorders. *Journal of Communication Disorders, 32,* 223–245.

Otomo, K., & Stoel-Gammon, C. (1992). The acquisition of unrounded vowels in English. *Journal of Speech and Hearing Research, 35,* 604–616.

Owens, R. E. (1994). *Language development: An introduction* (4th ed.). Allyn & Bacon.

Pollock, K. E. (2002). Identification of vowel errors: Methodological issues and preliminary data from the Memphis Vowel Project. In M. J. Ball, & F. E. Gibbon (Eds.), *Vowel disorders* (pp. 83–113). Butterworth Heinemann.

Pollock, K. E., & Berni, M. C. (2003). Incidence of non-rhotic vowel errors in children: Data from the Memphis Vowel Project. *Clinical Linguistics and Phonetics, 17,* 393–401.

Porter, J. H., & Hodson, B. W. (2001). Collaborating to obtain phonological acquisition data for local schools. *Language, Speech, and Hearing Services in Schools, 32,* 165–171.

Preisser, D. A., Hodson, B. W., & Paden, E. P. (1988). Developmental phonology: 18–29 months. *Journal of Speech and Hearing Disorders, 53,* 125–130.

Robb, M. P., & Bleile, K. M. (1994). Consonant inventories of young children from 8 to 25 months. *Clinical Linguistics and Phonetics, 8,* 295–320.

Robbins, J., & Klee, T. (1987). Clinical assessment of oropharyngeal motor development in young children. *Journal of Speech and Hearing Disorders, 52,* 271–277.

Roberts, J. E., Burchinal, M., & Footo, M. M. (1990). Phonological process decline from 2;6 to 8 years. *Journal of Communication Disorders, 23,* 205–217.

Ruben, R. J. (1997). A time frame of critical/sensitive periods of language development. *Acta Otolaryngology, 117,* 202–205.

Selby, J. C., Robb, M. P., & Gilbert, H. R. (2000). Normal vowel articulations between 15 and 36 months of age. *Clinical Linguistics and Phonetics, 14,* 255–266.

Shriberg, L. D. (1993). Four new speech and prosody-voice measures for genetics research and other studies in developmental phonological disorders. *Journal of Speech and Hearing Research, 36,* 105–140.

Shriberg, L. D., & Kwiatkowski, J. (1982). Phonological disorders III: A procedure for assessing severity of involvement. *Journal of Speech and Hearing Disorders, 47,* 256–270.

Shriberg, L. D., Kwiatkowski, J., & Gruber, F. A. (1994). Developmental phonological disorders II: Short-term speech-sound normalisation. *Journal of Speech and Hearing Research, 37,* 1127–1150.

Smit, A. B. (1993a). Phonologic error distributions in the Iowa-Nebraska articulation norms project: Consonant singletons. *Journal of Speech and Hearing Research, 36,* 533–547.

Smit, A. B. (1993b). Phonologic error distributions in the Iowa-Nebraska articulation norms project: Word-initial consonant clusters. *Journal of Speech and Hearing Research, 36,* 931–947.

Smit, A. B., Hand, L., Frelinger, J. J., Bernthal, J. E., & Bird, A. (1990). The Iowa articulation norms project and its Nebraska replication. *Journal of Speech and Hearing Disorders, 55,* 779–798.

Stark, R. E., Bernstein, L. E., & Demorest, M. E. (1993). Vocal communication in the first 18 months of life. *Journal of Speech and Hearing Research, 36,* 548–558.

Stoel-Gammon, C. (1985). Phonetic inventories, 15–24 months: A longitudinal study. *Journal of Speech and Hearing Research, 28,* 505–512.

Stoel-Gammon, C. (1987). Phonological skills of 2-year-olds. *Language, Speech, and Hearing Services in Schools, 18,* 323–329.

Vihman, M. (1988). Early phonological development. In J. Bernthal & N. Bankson (Eds), *Articulation and phonological disorders* (2nd ed.) Williams & Wilkins.

Watson, M. M., & Scukanec, G. P. (1997a). Phonological changes in the speech of two-year olds: A longitudinal investigation. *Infant-Toddler Intervention, 7,* 67–77.

Watson, M. M., & Scukanec, G. P. (1997b). Profiling the phonological abilities of 2-year-olds: A longitudinal investigation. *Child Language Teaching and Therapy, 13,* 3–14.

Williams, A. L., & Elbert, M. (2003). A prospective longitudinal study of phonological development in late talkers. *Language, Speech, and Hearing Services in Schools, 34,* 138–153.

References

Alt, M., Figueroa, C. R., Mettler, H. M., Evans-Reitz, N., & Erikson, J. A. (2021). A vocabulary acquisition and usage for Late Talkers treatment efficacy study: The effect of input utterance length and identification of responder profiles. *Journal of Speech, Language, and Hearing Research, 64*(4), 1235–1255. https://doi.org/10.1044/2020_JSLHR-20-00525

American Speech-Language-Hearing Association. (2007). *Directory of speech-language pathology assessment instruments: II. Articulation/phonology assessment: Children.* Author.

Bowen, C. (2003). *Caroline Bowen: Speech-Language Pathologist.* http://www.slpsite.com

Capone Singleton, N. (2018). Late talkers: Why the wait-and-see approach is outdated. *Pediatric Clinics of North America, 65*(1),13–29. https://doi.org/10.1016/j.pcl.2017.08.018

Carter, J. A., Lees, J. A., Murira, G. M., Gona, J., Neville, B. G. R., & Newton, C. R. J. C. (2005). Issues in the development of cross-cultural assessments of speech and language for children. *International Journal of Language & Communication Disorders, 40*(4), 385–401.

Cronin, A., McLeod, S., & Verdon, S. (2020). Holistic communication assessment for young children with cleft palate using the International Classification of Functioning, Disability and Health: Children and Youth. *Language, Speech, and Hearing Services in Schools, 51*(4), 914–938. https://doi.org/10.1044/2020_LSHSS-19-00122

Crowe, K., & McLeod, S. (2020). Children's English consonant acquisition in the United States: A review. *American Journal of Speech-Language Pathology.* http://doi.org/101044/2020_AJSLP-19-0018

Davis, B., & Bedore, L. (2013). *An emergence approach to speech acquisition: Doing and knowing.* Psychology Press.

Dyson, A. (1988). Phonetic inventories of 2-year-old children. *Journal of Speech and Hearing Disorders, 53,* 89–93.

Fenson, L., Dale, P. S., Reznick, J., Thal, D., Bates, E., Hartung, J., Pethick, S., & Reilly, J. (1993). *MacArthur Communicative Development Inventories (CDIs).* Paul H. Brookes Publishing Co.

Fenson, L., Marchman, V. A., Thal, D., Dale, P. S., Reznick, J. S., & Bates, E. (2007). *MacArthur-Bates Communicative Development Inventories (CDIs): User's Guide and technical manual* (2nd ed.). Paul H. Brookes Publishing Co.

Fenson, L., Marchman, V. A., Thal, D., Dale, P. S., Reznick, J. S., & Bates, E. (2007). *MacArthur-Bates Communicative Development Inventories (CDIs) Words and Sentences.* Paul H. Brookes Publishing Co.

Ferguson, C., & Farwell, C. (1975). Words and sounds in early language acquisition. *Language, 51,* 39–49.

Flipsen, Jr., P. (2006). Measuring the intelligibility of conversational speech in children. *Clinical Linguistics & Phonetics, 20*(4), 303–312.

Fudala, J. B. (2017). *Arizona 4: Arizona Articulation and Phonology Scale, Fourth Revision.* Western Psychological Services.

Goldman, R., & Fristoe, M. (2015). *Goldman-Fristoe Test of Articulation, Third Edition.* AGS Publishing/ Pearson.

Hodges, R., Baker, E., Munro, N., & McGregor, K. (2016). Responses made by late talkers and typically developing toddlers during speech assessments. *International Journal of Speech-Language Pathology, 19*(6), 587–600, https://doi.org/10.1080/17549507.2016.1221452

Hodson, B. W. (2004). *HAPP-3: Hodson Assessment of Phonological Patterns–Third Edition.* PRO-ED.

Individuals with Disabilities Education Improvement Act (IDEA) of 2004, PL 108-446, 20 U.S.C. §§ 1400 *et seq.*

Kwiatkowski, J., & Shriberg, L. (1983, November). *Classification studies of developmental phonologic disorders: Evidence for subgroups.* Paper presented at the Annual Convention of the American Speech-Language-Hearing Association, Cincinnati.

Marchman, V. A., Dale, P. S., & Fenson, L. (2023). *MacArthur-Bates Communicative Development Inventories (CDIs)* (3rd ed.). Paul H. Brookes Publishing Co.

Masterson, J., & Bernhardt, B. H. (2001). *CAPES: Computerized Articulation & Phonology Evaluation System*. Psychological Corporation.

McGregor, K. K., Williams, D., Hearst, S., & Johnson, A. C. (1997). The use of contrastive analysis in distinguishing difference from disorder: A tutorial. *American Journal of Speech-Language Pathology, 6,* 45–56.

McIntosh, B., & Dodd, B. (2008). Two-year-olds' phonological acquisition: Normative data. *International Journal of Speech-Language Pathology, 10*(6), 460–469.

McLeod, S., & Bleile K. (2003, Nov.) *Neurological and developmental foundations of speech acquisition* [handout]. Invited seminar at the annual convention of the American Speech-Language-Hearing Association, Philadelphia, PA, United States.

McLeod, S., & Crowe, K. (2018). Children's consonant acquisition in 27 languages: A cross-linguistic review. *American Journal of Speech-Language Pathology, 27*(4), 1546–1571. https://doi.org/10.1044/2018 _AJSLP-17-0100

McLeod, S., Margetson, K., Wang, C., Tran, V., Verdon, S., White, K., & Phạm, B. (2021). Speech acquisition within a 3-generation Vietnamese-English family: The influence of maturation and ambient phonology. *Clinical Linguistics and Phonetics*. Advance online publication. https://doi.org/10.1080 /02699206.2020.1862915

McLeod, S., Verdon, S., & International Expert Panel on Multilingual Children's Speech. (2017). Tutorial: Speech assessment for multilingual children who do not speak the same language(s) as the speech-language pathologist. *American Journal of Speech-Language Pathology, 26*(3), 691–708. https://doi.org /10.1044/2017_AJSLP-15-0161

McManus, B. M., Richardson, Z., Schenkman, M., Murphy, N., Everhart, R. M., Hambidge, S., & Morrato, E. (2020). Child characteristics and early intervention referral and receipt of services: A retrospective cohort study. *BMC Pediatric, 20*(84). https://doi.org/10.1186/s12887-020-1965-x

Miccio, A., & Elbert, M. (1996). Enhancing stimulability: A treatment program. *Journal of Communication Disorders, 29,* 335–351.

Miccio, A., & Williams, A. L. (2021). Stimulability Approach (pp. 279–304). In A. L. Williams, S. McLeod, & R. J. McCauley (Eds.), *Interventions for speech sound disorders in children* (2nd ed.). Paul H. Brookes Publishing Co.

Morrison, C. M., Chappell, T. D., Ellis, A. W. (1997). Age of acquisition norms for a large set of object names and their relation to adult estimates and other variables. *Quarterly Journal of Experimental Psychology, 50*(3), 528–559.

Munro, N., Baker, E., Masso, S., Carson, L. Lee, T., Wong, A. M.-Y., & Stokes, S. F. (2021). Vocabulary acquisition and usage for late talkers treatment: Effect on expressive vocabulary and phonology. *Journal of Speech, Language, and Hearing Research, 64,* 2682-2697. https://doi.org/10.1044/2021_JSLHR-20-00680

Olswang, L., Stoel-Gammon, C., Coggins, T., & Carpenter, R. (1987). *Assessing prelinguistic and early linguistic behaviors in developmentally young children*. University of Washington Press.

Paul, R. (1991). Profiles of toddlers with slow expressive language development. *Topics in Language Disorders, 11,* 1–13.

Paul, R. (1993). Patterns of development in late talkers: Preschool years. *Journal of Childhood Communication Disorders, 15,* 7–14.

Paul, R., & Jennings, P. (1992). Phonological behaviors in toddlers with slow expressive language development. *Journal of Speech and Hearing Research, 35,* 99–107.

Paul, R., Spangle-Looney, S., & Dahm, P. (1991). Communication and socialization skills at age 2 and 3 in "late talking" children. *Journal of Speech and Hearing Research, 34,* 858–865.

Peña, E., & Quinn, R. (1997). Task familiarity: Effects on the test performance of Puerto Rican and African American children. *Language Speech and Hearing Services in Schools, 28,* 323–332.

Peña, E., Quinn, R., & Iglesias, A. (1992). The application of dynamic methods to language assessment: A nonbiased procedure. *Journal of Special Education, 26,* 269–280.

Preisser, D., Hodson, B., & Paden, E. (1988). Developmental phonology: 18–29 months. *Journal of Speech and Hearing Disorders, 53,* 125–130.

Rescorla, L., & Dale, P. S. (2013). *Late talkers: Language development, interventions, and outcomes*. Paul H. Brookes Publishing Co.

Rescorla, L., & Ratner, N. B. (1996). Phonetic profiles of toddlers with specific expressive language impairment (SLI-E). *Journal of Speech and Hearing Research, 39,* 153–165.

Scherer, N., Kaiser, A., & Frey, J. (2021). Enhanced milieu teaching with phonological emphasis (pp. 305–336). In A. L. Williams, S. McLeod, & R. J. McCauley (Eds.), *Interventions for speech sound disorders in children* (2nd ed.). Paul H. Brookes Publishing Co.

Scherer, N., Williams, A. L., Stoel-Gammon, C., & Kaiser, A. (2012). Assessment of single-word production for children under three years of age: Comparison of children with and without cleft palate. *International Journal of Otolaryngology, 2012,* 724214. https://doi.org/10.1155/2012/724214

Schwartz, R. G., & Leonard, L. B. (1982). Do children pick and choose? An examination of phonological selection and avoidance in early lexical acquisition. *Journal of Child Language, 9*(2), 319–336.

Smit, A. B. (1986). Ages of speech sound acquisition: Comparisons and critiques of several normative studies. *Language, Speech, and Hearing Services in Schools, 17,* 175–186.

Smit, A. B., Hand, L., Freilinger, J. J., Bernthal, J. E., & Bird, A. (1990). The Iowa Articulation Norms Project and its Nebraska replication. *Journal of Speech and Hearing Disorders, 55,* 779–798.

Sosa, A. V., & Stoel-Gammon, C. (2012). Lexical and phonological effects in early word production. *Journal of Speech, Language, and Hearing Research, 55*(2), 596–608. https://doi.org/10.1044/1092 -4388(2011/10-0113)

Shriberg, L. D., & Kwiatkowski, J. (1982). Phonological Disorders III: A procedure for assessing severity of involvement. *Journal of Speech and Hearing Disorders, 47,* 256–270.

Stoel-Gammon, C. (1985). Phonetic inventories, 15–24 months: A longitudinal study. *Journal of Speech and Hearing Research, 28,* 505–512.

Stoel-Gammon, C. (1987). Phonological skills of two-year-olds. *Language, Speech, and Hearing Services in Schools, 18,* 323–329.

Stoel-Gammon, C. (1988). Evaluation of phonological skills in preschool children. *Seminars in Speech and Language, 9*(1), 15–25.

Stoel-Gammon, C. (1989). Prespeech and early speech development of two late talkers. *First Language, 9,* 207–224.

Stoel-Gammon, C. (1991). Normal and disordered phonology in two-year-olds. *Topics in Language Disorders, 11,* 21–32.

Stoel-Gammon, C. (1994). Measuring phonology in babble and speech. *Clinics in Communication Disorders, 4*(1), 1–11.

Stoel-Gammon, C. (2010). The Word Complexity Measure: Description and application to developmental phonology and disorders. *Clinical Linguistics and Phonetics 24,* 271–282.

Stoel-Gammon, C. (2011). Relationships between lexical and phonological development in young children. *Journal of Child Language, 38,* 1–34.

Stoel-Gammon, C., & Cooper, J. A. (1984). Patterns of early lexical and phonological development. *Journal of Child Language, 11*(2), 247–271.

Stoel-Gammon, C., & Dunn, C. (1985). *Normal and disordered phonology in children.* PRO-ED.

Stoel-Gammon, C., & Stone, J. (1991). Assessing phonology in young children. *Clinics in Communication Disorders, 2,* 25–39.

Stoel-Gammon, C., & Williams, A. L. (2013). Early phonological development: Creating an assessment test. *Clinical Linguistics & Phonetics, 27,* 278–286.

Stokes, S. F. (2014). The impact of phonological neighborhood density on typical and atypical emerging lexicons. *Journal of Child Language, 41,* 634-756.

Watson, M., & Scukanec, G. (1997). Profiling the phonological abilities of 2-year-olds: A longitudinal study. *Child Language Teaching and Therapy, 13,* 31–50.

Williams, A., & Elbert, M. (2003). A prospective longitudinal study of phonological development in late talkers. *Language, Speech and Hearing Services in Schools, 34,* 138–153.

Williams, A., McLeod, S., & McCauley, R. (Eds.). (2021). *Interventions for speech sound disorders in children* (2nd ed.). Paul H. Brookes Publishing Co.

Williams, A. L., & Stoel-Gammon, C. (2016, Nov.). *Identification of speech-language disorders in toddlers.* Invited seminar at the annual convention of the American Speech-Language-Hearing Association, Philadelphia, PA, United States.

Index

Note: Page numbers followed by *f*, *b*, and *t* indicate figures, boxes, and tables, respectively.